ESSENTIAL
NURSERY MANAGEMENT

ESSENTIAL
NURSERY MANAGEMENT

Susan Hay

BAILLIÈRE TINDALL
London Philadelphia Sydney Tokyo Toronto

Baillière Tindall   24–28 Oval Road
London NW1 7DX

The Curtis Center
Independence Square West
Philadelphia, PA 19106–3399, USA

Harcourt Brace & Company
55 Horner Avenue
Toronto, Ontario, M8Z 4X6, Canada

Harcourt Brace & Company, Australia
30–52 Smidmore Street
Marrickville
NSW 2204, Australia

Harcourt Brace & Company, Japan
Ichibancho Central Building
22–1 Ichibancho
Chiyoda-ku, Tokyo 102, Japan

Photographs © Maggie Murray/Format

A catalogue record for this book is available from the British Library

ISBN 0-7020-2044-3

Typeset by Selwood Typesetters, Frome, Somerset
Printed and bound in Great Britain by WBC Book Manufacturers Ltd,
Bridgend, Mid Glamorgan.

Contents

Foreword

There is an unusual degree of agreement across the political divide on the importance of nursery education. It is widely accepted that children who have benefited from nursery education make better progress in the later stages of education and are less likely to be disruptive or become 'delinquent'.

There is much less agreement, however, as to what nursery education should involve and how it should be delivered. Should it be available for three-year olds or only for four-year olds; how much and in what way should parents be involved; to what extent should it be entrusted to specially trained professionals?

These issues are discussed in this book but there are two statements which can categorically be made: good nursery education should include both appropriate education and high quality care and it cannot be done on the cheap.

Essentially the money put into nursery education is not primarily the payment of the costs of a useful service. It is an investment, and a long term investment at that. The harvest of better educated and better adjusted men and women will not begin to be reaped for at least fifteen years. But it will then be a harvest that will benefit both the individual and society and it will be paid in both economic and social coin. Today our greatest economic disadvantage in world competition is our long tail of uneducated and untrained people, the major cause of high unemployment. If, as is widely accepted, nursery education can substantially increase the numbers of the educated and trained, the economic case is won. The maladjusted individual, teenager or adult, who swells the crime figures bringing misery to many law-abiding citizens also swells the numbers in our overcrowded prisons. Since a week in prison costs at least four hundred pounds, if nursery education reduces these numbers, the economic case once again is made.

Nor must it be overlooked that it is not only the children who benefit in nursery education. If the lone parent can leave their child in a nursery, they are more able to obtain work to support themselves. The highly qualified professional woman or experienced specialist also stands to gain and society gains from her work. Many such women are straining themselves in an attempt

to be simultaneously the perfect mother and the perfect professional. Often they are dogged by a continuous sense of guilt and
many just give up the battle. For such women the knowledge that
really high level nursery provision is available can make all the
difference. But it must be high level. Susan Hay describes here the
conditions under which such provision can be made and the priorities which managers of such provision should establish to meet
this complex and serious challenge. Cut price nursery education
cannot deliver these valuable goods. "Penny wise, pound foolish."

Baroness Seear PC
Deputy Leader of the Liberal Democrats
House of Lords

Preface

Management is about ensuring that every moment of everyone's time is invested shrewdly – that is, in the most effective way possible. It is about ensuring that something more worthwhile could not have been done in place of what was in fact done: no waste, clear focusing, pinpointing, routines to ensure smooth operations, no more people than necessary.

The nurturing and education of very young children does not easily recall such skills and attitudes.

To what extent can 'normal' management approaches help, in the endeavour to provide good early years' services? This question requires us to look at who the stakeholders are in early years' services. There are a number of them – all with differing priorities and different reasons for being involved:

- the parents, whose overriding concern is to achieve the best start in life for their child;
- the child, who must settle, enjoy for its own value his or her time at nursery, and who must benefit from the development and learning opportunities;
- the local authority acting within its statutory duty to ensure provision is safe and sure;
- the staff who seek a rewarding role;
- the driving force, who may own the business or lead the voluntary organisation, whose passion is responsible for the existence of the provision, and who may also manage the nursery;
- the shareholders in a larger organisation who will wish to see a return on their investment;
- developers who are concerned that the 'amenity' they have accommodated makes sense in terms of their real property interests; and
- employers who will be monitoring the impact of a nursery provision on their workforce.

This is probably not an exhaustive list, but it serves to illustrate the range of priorities that the main stakeholders will have. It follows that the services we provide must also differ, in order that they respect and include all stakeholders' interests and emphases. We cannot and should not deny such differences.

However, we can and should find ways of holding on to both sets of essential values: values of good childcare and values of good management.

This book is essentially a discussion of the 'non-negotiable' aspects of early years' services management. How can we resolve the impossible daily dilemma of quality versus costs? How can we ensure that services of quality are delivered within a planned management framework, one that allows them to be stable, permanent and to thrive?

Not one of the very different stakeholders' interests is served by lack of management: there is neither a future in charging so little for a service that, despite everyone being able to afford it, costs are not covered; nor any in charging so much that an excellent service can be ensured yet for most parents is prohibitively expensive.

A balance has to be struck – a balance you can live with. This is the aspect that is hard for those involved, and much harder – and much scarier – than for those with most other types of small business. Here, the foundations of early learning are being cast, the life chances the young child will have are to an extent determined by the quality of early years' experience.

This book aims to link the components of good management with the components of good childcare. I have attempted to take up from where most professional training for early years' practitioners leaves off, drawing heavily on my own experience of running a group of nurseries. I am indebted to all of the recognised thinkers in both fields and have drawn, in particular, from Charles Handy, Bob Garratt and Patrick Whittaker on management, and from Peter Moss, Peter Elfer and Margy Whalley on early years.

It was tempting to call the book 'What They Don't Teach on Early Years' Courses', not by way of criticism but in recognising that practice has changed dramatically and we must all learn from those who are in management positions now.

With special thanks to my 'steering group': Alistair, the best intuitive, creative and reluctant manager I know; Neil, now 17, who had a 'mixed' early years' experience; Holly, now 11, who had no option but her mother; and Adam, 7, who has recently completed his 'career' at my own Floral Place Nursery.

The book is for all those who want to sustain a good childcare business, and motivate others into doing the same.

Acknowledgements

All photographs were taken at Nurseryworks Ltd nurseries in London and are used with thanks to children, parents and staff of Broadgate Nursery, Floral Place Nursery, Billets Corner Nursery, Dulwich Nursery and Alperton Nursery.

Dedication

The book is dedicated to all the staff of my own company Nurseryworks Ltd from whom I have learned so much about young children, young adults and a young business.

Susan Hay, Managing Director of
Susan Hay Associates Limited and Nurseryworks Limited
Childcare Planning and Nursery Management

Introduction

Angela Rumbold's *Starting with Quality* (1990) said: 'For the early years in education, the process of education – how children are encouraged to learn, is as important as, and inseparable from the content – what they learn.'

This book is not about young children as learners, or the content of learning, but about the context in which they develop and the conditions that are conducive to delivering this entitlement.

Vernon and Smith, in *Day Nurseries at a Crossroads* (1994), observed: 'One of the casualties of the current system of financing nurseries is that insufficient attention is paid to the management needs of running a nursery. The day to day demands of running a nursery should not be underestimated, and require a high degree of flexibility and adaptability on the part of the nursery manager. However, many nursery managers seem to be drawn (sometimes quite unwittingly) into substantial "hands on" working with children, leaving them limited time for more strategic matters, the general running of the nursery, the supervision of staff and developing practice.'

In this book I have taken this observation a step further, and suggested that, rather than 'sometimes quite unwittingly', new managers have no option but to fall back into being the best team member, as no one has given *them* any support or guidance in fulfilling their new role of manager. Nursery managers can obtain a great deal of help to do their 'old' job better; to reflect on and think strategically about all the issues involved, from undertaking further qualifications and from local authority advisers. However, many are not aware of the new concerns of a manager; you cannot recognise what you do not know.

What I hope the book will achieve is the fostering of a new attitude towards self-appraisal – but not of the individual so much as the practising unit as a whole; i.e. the *nursery's performance and development plan,* for which the manager is responsible.

Angela Rumbold said that self-appraisal, with the aim of enhancing confidence and professionalism, lies at the heart of efforts to improve quality.

Appraisal systems that focus on the needs of the individual are an important part of good employment practice, but they are only one cog in the wheel of continuous improvement in the nursery service as a whole. The *Investor in People* scheme (Chapter 4) provides a model for 'total quality management' when applied to a nursery setting. Recognising that quality of staff and quality of service are almost indiscriminate, it provides a means of proving that attending to the development of staff makes good business sense. This is helpful, and relevant, when between 50% and 70% of all fees received will be expended on staff. And it is perhaps more pertinent – given that quality of service is so inextricably linked with the quality of staff – than broader quality measurement standards.

The new registration and inspection system that was introduced by the Children Act was designed to safeguard minimum standards whilst promoting a quality service, but without discouraging service developments by overly tight requirements. These aims have confused some nursery providers who find it difficult to differentiate between the standards required for registration and those that are concerned with good practice. According to the Social Services Inspectorate, nursery providers are more accepting of the changes brought about by the Children Act when the local authority has been quite clear about the difference between its registration requirements and the standards it would like to see achieved to provide quality care. The providers then know where they stand.

I do not repeat the Children Act requirements here, or put myself in the position of a local authority inspector; rather I try to consider another level of quality standard, the one that you want to achieve, every moment of every day, despite staff absences, moody children and pressurised parents.

In *Day Nurseries at a Crossroads* (Vernon and Smith 1994), the National Children's Bureau suggested that it was time for an analysis of management functions in nurseries and, in particular, of management roles. Angela Rumbold referred to the need for 'clear management structures' back in 1990.

My concern here is that management is not seen as a separate function, rather one that is integrated into the nursery service as a whole. This would be described as the 'horizontal approach', with a management attitude permeating all aspects of the nursery service – in the same way, if you like, as care and education of young children are inseparable.

As to the future, again Rumbold carried some important pointers:

- how to establish or improve links between the practitioner's own organisation and other local services for the under-fives;
- whether there is scope for coordinating with other service aspects such as admission policies, liaison with families and schools, observation and record-keeping arrangements;
- a new approach on the part of those responsible for existing arrangements which impede collaboration, i.e. developing partnerships.

Practitioners were called on by Rumbold to set clear quality objectives, and regularly to review standards achieved; to consider how best to involve parents and to spend time on their own professional development; to reconsider the real barriers to entry into the profession. When I set out on this book project, I had not appreciated how much of the work would relate to providing some suggestions for the practical application of Rumbold's work.

- Chapter 1 looks at the nature of nursery management. How do we approach things differently as a manager and on what does developing such an approach rely?
- Chapter 2 looks at the important management issues and how we can deal with these effectively.
- Chapter 3 looks at what is involved in leading a team; how it affects you and others.
- Chapter 4 looks at staff as an investment; how we find them and how we foster their development.
- Chapter 5 looks at the manager as nursery ambassador; how to articulate what the nursery offers, and approaches to addressing the concerns of parents.
- Chapter 6 looks at the importance of working to a plan; treating the nursery as a small business, and dealing with finance.
- Chapter 7 looks at how a nursery moves forward; how it reviews its service and adapts to change.

In summary, I have attempted to set out the issues that have required special attention and principles that have guided me, with examples of what I have found to work in my own setting. I have drawn heavily on my own experience, rather than academic texts, although further reading is recommended. What is here has worked for me and my company, which currently runs five nurseries in London and is developing more. I have not prescribed how you should run your individual nursery, for your children and your parents.

1

Who is a Manager and What is Management?

- Management and Leadership

- Fit to Manage in the Eyes of Others

- Manager's Rite of Passage

- Maturing as a Manager

- Are Nursery Managers Born or are They Made?

Management and Leadership

People who are selected or are identified as nursery managers are used to managing. The care and education of young children inevitably requires organisational skills, setting expectations of behaviour, maintaining standards, evaluating outcomes – all the issues normally covered in professional qualifications and training for nursery nurses and teachers. However, this innate experience does not seem to translate easily when it comes to applying it to the nursery as a whole. Here, managers develop the skills they need to fulfil their role, for themselves, often in an isolated, unsupported environment. For some reason, there is no recognisable management structure that could advance the professionalisation of nursery managers as it is perceived by others. In the words of Patrick Whittaker (1995), 'ask yourself whether you have the skills to run British Gas, and ask yourself whether the Chairman of British Gas could run your nursery? And who outside the nursery world would recognise the answer?'

Management of a nursery, in my view, encompasses both management as it is usually thought of, and leadership – which is generally believed to be something broader than management. Leaders are people who can influence the behaviour of others for the purpose of achieving a goal. Leaders possess a special set of rather baffling qualities which enable them to persuade others to do what the leader wants because they want to do it. Leaders can balance concern for the task, for quality and for efficiency, with equal concern for the people they work with and the relationships between them.

Managers are understood to be concerned with routine and focusing on the present. Their actions are usually dominated by issues of continuity and stability. The differences between leadership and management have been noted by Hodgkinson (1991):

- leadership is an art whereas management is a science;
- leadership is focused on policy whereas management is concerned with execution;
- leadership is concerned with values whereas management looks at facts;
- leadership is generalist, management is specialist;
- leadership uses broad strategies rather than management's specific tactics;

- leadership is concerned with philosophy rather than action;
- leaders are reflective, managers are active;
- leaders are concerned with human resources whereas managers are concerned with material resources;
- leaders focus on deliberation, managers on detail.

In most nursery settings the manager is indeed required also to be the leader. The financial constraints of having two people at this level usually require both roles to be filled by the same individual and it is probably only within the larger nursery groups that you begin to see the distinction emerge. The syndrome of having to deal with both roles is often described by management consultants as management of the 'important versus the immediate', where important refers to those big value-based issues with which a leader is concerned, vying for time with the manager's need to respond to day-to-day problems that constantly arise.

While it is true that in order to be an effective leader you need to be an efficient manager, management skills do not equate with leadership skills – they are much wider. Also, although having highly developed management skills will probably allow you to create time for leadership functions as well, having poorly developed management skills will inevitably prohibit attention being paid to leadership functions. This book uses 'management' to describe the combination of leadership and management required in nursery settings.

Illustrating how leadership and management come together for those in early years' services, Gillian Rodd (1994) lists the essential characteristics for the job:

- *Curiosity* (interest in learning)
- *Candour* (open to public scrutiny and willingness to speak the truth)
- *Courtesy* (respect and dignity for others)
- *Courage* (willingness to take risks, dare, make mistakes)
- *Compassion* (creating trust and empathy).

Fit to Manage in the Eyes of Others

The National Children's Bureau's (NCB) *Guidelines for Good Practice in Group Daycare* (1991) describes the management responsibility as:

- ensuring that the nursery is operating smoothly;
- responding to the needs of parents, children and staff;
- being open to suggestions for development.

These three points encapsulate the essential needs for:

- policies and procedures to be understood and followed;
- staff to be empowered to make decisions that are flexible to changing needs;
- recognition that new knowledge and new ideas need to be continuously assessed and incorporated into practice.

Each of these three concepts requires the manager to learn continuously: from mistakes, from other people, and from other ways of going about running a nursery.

When we combine the need for learning, and the need to develop directing ability, we create the idea of the *learning leader*. This is a more appropriate title for the person responsible for ensuring that the NCB Guidelines are met; that the service is managed in a way appropriate to a changing profile of children, a changing profile of parents, a changing staff team, new thought on how children develop, and new legislation.

The first stage is to learn from what is actually going on in your nursery. If we consider the circumstances that led to recent tragedies such as the sinking of the Herald of Free Enterprise, the King's Cross Underground fire, the Clapham Junction rail crash, and the Hillsborough Stadium collapse, they all become more disturbing as evidence showed that the knowledge necessary to help avoid the disasters already lay within the organisations. But there was no system for sharing the knowledge, no means of fully learning from previous mistakes. Information must be allowed to flow to that part of the organisation with the responsibility for taking preventive action.

In a nursery setting, when information does not flow freely and openly in the interests of children and parents, this can be characterised as 'oh I thought she was doing that' or 'if only you'd told me that earlier' – all contributing to destroying cooperation, encouraging buck passing and undermining instructions.

The first step for a new manager, then, is to create or review the *learning system* by which the nursery can become both more effective and more efficient. This combines the written policies and procedures, and routines for review and evaluation of practice. Both these issues are dealt with in Chapter 2. Local authorities have a specific view, for the purpose of registering a nursery under the Children Act 1989, of what makes a manager 'fit' *and this will need to be ascertained as a starting point.*

Manager's Rite of Passage

The second step is for the manager to go through an important rite of passage:

> *'You are now so valuable to us, that you must leave the day-to-day operation of the organisation, and have time and space to think about how effective we are in relation to the changing entitlements and needs of children and parents, what the future of those changes might mean, how we can position ourselves strategically and how we can create a system of rapid learning so that we may keep up with those changes.'*

Most nursery managers have received little training for their present job. This puts them on a par with their equivalents in most other walks of life. Rarely is there time or money budgeted for the leader, however strong the commitment to training further down the line.

A further block to reaching the real manager role derives from the earlier point: because no one has taught managers to manage, and because many have reached the managerial position because they are the best at what they do – as the senior member of the team – they get hooked on their old operational role (see Case Study 1). In the absence of any transition or training, it is not thought to be legitimate to develop a new role. This tends to manifest itself in firefighting the *immediate,* rather than thinking about the *important.* 'This Action Fixated rather than Action Learning approach is the curse of management', says Bob Garratt (1990).

Having committed yourself to the notion of action-learning, and having considered what is necessary to change your own mind from one of operative to manager, it is time to deal with the development of others. If you are to provide a consistently good service then all staff must be empowered to make decisions that provide parents and children with solutions to their needs.

It is necessary for the manager to coach, counsel and train

Case Study 1

Manager slipping back into old role

Caroline had been promoted to manage a new nursery set up by the company she had worked with as a Deputy Coordinator of another of their nurseries. In the new nursery the focus was to be on receiving prospective parents and selling places, and building a new staff team.

Caroline was supported by the company's Childcare Manager, Education Consultant and Managing Director. The nursery was planned to have a large baby unit, which would inevitably fill first, with children of parents working locally. Caroline had particular experience with babies and a wealth of knowledge of health and safety issues.

A reputation for offering a high-quality service for babies, which matched the needs of working parents, was quickly established. The parent group had high expectations, and being subjected to work pressures of their own were similarly demanding of staff. This need was in the main met by Caroline, who was understandably anxious that staff should not become anxious about responding to, very often, concerned and nervous first-time parents.

A pattern grew up of Caroline coping with the demands of parents, and other members of the team recognising that this was a special skill Caroline possessed. It also became the norm for Caroline herself to take a role in the baby unit if the staff were stretched or if a member of the team was absent. Parents became accustomed to her presence and confidence in the service was linked with her presence. For Caroline's part, she was doing what she did best: handling parents with great diplomacy and confidence, and caring for babies.

The baby unit, however, was the stated responsibility of a Senior Nursery Officer. When Caroline was present the Senior naturally stepped out of her own management role and referred to Caroline on decisions. Similarly, the rest of the team slipped back one rung.

The effect of Caroline's management style was two-fold: for herself, it meant that it was increasingly difficult to focus on the managerial issues that the manager is uniquely capable of undertaking – some of which were office-based, but not all – with the result that the company considered that she had not embraced the full responsibility of being the manager; for the Senior Nursery Officer it meant that she had limited opportunity to demonstrate her own strengths in the role.

others to do the same as you. These are the systems, provision and techniques of supervision, appraisal, staff meetings and in-service training (see Chapter 3).

How then does the whole nursery move forward? On top of the expectations we have of ourselves, based on the service we purport to offer, what of the ever-increasing expectations of others? Today's excellence is merely tomorrow's standard, and never is this more true than in the nursery world. If you *know* that children thrive under certain conditions, in certain environments, with certain principles in place, how can anyone accept second best? In this industry, there are no 'special purchases' or 'B grades'.

Embracing change and the turbulence it can cause requires maturity in a manager. Faced with the moving target of *quality childcare*, change is part and parcel of everyday nursery life. The tools that the nursery manager requires here are ones of quality assurance, sound practice, consultation.

As a team member, you are a technical specialist – a nursery nurse or teacher. As a manager you are a generalist – knowing enough about every aspect of the nursery to give direction and support. Rather than responding to the instructions and advice of others, as a manager you need to anticipate what instructions and advice others will need.

Maturing as a Manager

'My family was delighted, my friends were delighted if a little envious, and my staff thought that it was great that one of us had made it. The only problem was that after a few months I felt totally inadequate, became depressed and dreamt only of getting out, or back to the stability of my old job.'

This is typical of comments I hear each day from nursery managers who have 'made it' through to the top of the nursery organisational tree. Why is it that at the very moment of apparent career success things seem to start going wrong, or cease to be at least enjoyable? Are people always promoted to their level of incompetence?

In my experience the majority of people called on to lead their organisations think this is so – and they are unhappy about it.

They feel cheated at the last hurdle, because they have little if any help to get into their new role.

The organisation of most nurseries is that of a 'flat pyramid' – a team of nursery staff work with a manager and it is usual for the manager to have come from the team, as this move represents a promotional opportunity in an organisation where few exist. As a member of the team the individual has probably worked to a well-defined job description, with clearly identified responsibilities and tasks. Suddenly, from this position as a single-function team member, you are asked to become a 'learning leader' (Garratt 1990). We talk a lot about the function of nurseries as facilitating the 'maturation' of young children, but what of the process of developing maturity in a job?

This process can be viewed as having six stages (Figure 1). *Induction* is a stage that is handled well in nurseries and involves introducing a newcomer to all aspects of 'the way we do things around here'. *Inclusion* is the second stage needed to mature in a job. This is a more subtle concept and rarely managed well – it is the opposite of 'being left to sink or swim' and is about being accepted in your role by colleagues. It is about personality and behaviour and conventions rather than technical ability and experience. People are rarely selected on such criteria, yet it is on these abilities that you will be included in – or excluded from – a working team. In order that acceptance or rejection is not left to the

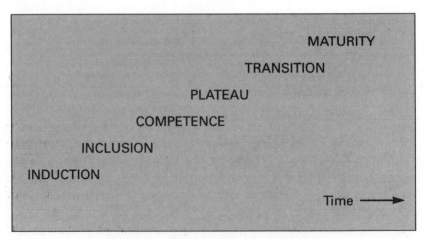

Figure 1. The process of development.

group, the new individual needs counselling and coaching and insight into what makes the group tick.

The third stage, *competence,* can be reached only if one has been fully included. Some would argue that, in being selected, the new recruit is *competent.* I would argue that competence is situational, and specific, and being competent in one setting does not necessarily mean that you will be competent in another, even though the role might be the same (i.e. nursery manager). Competence relies not only on abilities but on cooperation with others – inclusion in the group.

Once someone has been successfully inducted and included and has demonstrated their competence in the team, then they are ready to develop – bringing out what is within the individual to benefit the whole. This is often felt to be so alien to people's expectations of their job that it has to be made 'legitimate' before it can happen. Thus in the move from 'having a job' in the team to 'having a role' in the organisation, you are the kind of person that is valued by the organisation, and it is now time to contribute to how it will grow and how its culture will evolve. Through a process of self-development, an individual can add to their activities and expand their attitudes. This allows them to reset their personal targets and identify new challenges. Not only are they competent but they are also fulfilled, and able to bring their own special qualities to the job for which they are employed.

An individual reaches a *plateau* in terms of the development process when the individual, their boss and their staff are happy with the way things are going, and start resisting change. This can quickly lead to a stale working environment, or to the individual moving on! If *transition* is seen as a career change, then we are looking at promotion, redundancy, job rotation, etc.

The development process should apply to every working member of a team, but we are much better at looking after it for those who are not heading-up the team. Unless we focus on the needs and aspirations of the team leader, he or she will be limited in the leadership and managerial role: the person will keep their head down, search forever about what to do and how to do it, and begin to feel fairly wretched. It is difficult to say to your (junior) colleagues, 'Look, I am not becoming competent as your manager, I need some training.' In practice, overcoming this may mean that nursery managers must ensure that they provide this for themselves and form a network of external 'mentors'. Against the backcloth of the patchy and singular nursery industry, this feeling of isolation is often particularly acute.

The most common response, particularly if the resources of time and money for training are scarce, is to retreat into a position of comfort. To be precise, managers return to their old job, but this time unprofessionally. Relief is instant, as you slip back into old routines, language, and behaviour. But others are furious. What of the additional responsibility they had taken on when you were promoted? This knock-on effect continues down through the team, and can lead to people admitting that they are paid at a higher level than the job they actually do. The following are five specific ways for ensuring that such development blocks do not get in the way:

- Enable the manager to become involved in the review and for-mulation of policy, in order that it is not something simply received at the nursery level, from a management group on high, but rather that the nursery, through the manager, shares ownership of the policy change.
- Allow the manager time and space to review their strategic role, to take in and consider the impact of external changes on the nursery.
- Value and use the individual strengths of the manager, and supplement them with help in those areas in which they do not feel strong.
- Delegate problem-solving to staff team members.
- Accept that learning is continuous and free-flowing to wher-ever it is required.

Are Nursery Managers Born or are They Made?

There are three schools of thought on the making of managers: Do they possess certain innate traits that lend themselves to manage-ment? Do they behave with a certain style and have an approach that sets them apart from non-managers and enables them to exert influence over others? Or is it the situation in which they find themselves – the job that needs doing – that determines their need to manage?

Although personal characteristics can help, it is now generally recognised that management skills can be learned. It is also recognised that management potential can appear at any time in a career, leading to the notion that individuals can be capable of managing different situations at different stages in their lives. The demands of the situation and the characteristics of other people in the group will then determine the management skills required at that time and the most effective management style to adopt.

The nursery world in many countries is dominated by females. However, increasingly, and particularly as private sector provision accelerates, women are required to operate in the male world of finance, business and local government. Nursery managers need to understand and feel comfortable with male approaches to management at all levels, as well as dealing with their nursery community.

2

Focusing on the Task

- Balancing Needs and Expectations

- Decision-making

- Planning the Use of Resources

- Policies and Procedures

- External Pressure for Written Policies

- A Manual of Policies and Procedures

- Appendix

Balancing Needs and Expectations

A nursery manager is concerned with the needs of three main, separate, but interrelated groups of people. These are the children, their parents, and the staff who are employed. In addition there may be a Management Group or a Board of Management to consider.

The purpose for which the nursery is established is to provide a service for children. To do this well, both parents and staff must also be cared for and nurtured, but the service is and should remain the central focus of attention. Surprisingly, this idea can get lost, and a nursery can very soon become primarily concerned with meeting parents' requirements and aspirations. Or a nursery can start to revolve around the staff and their comfort, career development, and social life. Although all this is important, nothing is so critical as the confidence gained from knowing that everything you do as manager can be justified in terms of the service offered to children.

The very best situation would be one where both the quality of work (i.e. service (task) performance) and the quality of life (i.e. staff morale and parent satisfaction) are optimised. However, real life usually requires us to make choices, and I would argue that, where a choice has to be made, the service to children should not be allowed to suffer. A critical aspect of the manager's role is to raise awareness of the need, sometimes, to make such a choice, that the children's needs cannot be met in the best way if staff and parents achieve their preferences as well. So the manager must balance, as far as possible, these sometimes conflicting demands (see Case Study 2).

Striking the right balance will involve the manager in ensuring that:

- time is well used;
- the full abilities and contributions of the staff team are utilised;
- decisions are properly informed.

The issues I have found to require the most attention, in order to satisfy parents' expectations as well as children's entitlement, from a management perspective and whilst running our own nurseries over the last six years, are:

- teamwork;
- dealing with conflicts;
- selling the services of the nursery;
- working to a plan; and
- furthering the quality of service.

The roles and responsibilities involved in addressing these issues are dealt with later in Chapter 5.

Decision-making

Decision-making is part of everyday life in a nursery, and involves making choices. The quality of decisions made will affect the quality of the service provided, and it is the manager's responsibility to ensure that the best information available is at hand on which to base a decision. If decision-making is to be delegated in any part, then the manager must ensure that the individual to whom it is delegated is fully supported (see Chapter 4).

Available information will be consistent with the manager's experience: to what extent has a similar situation arisen before and how effective was the decision taken at that time? Equally important is the professional underpinning knowledge that the manager has to bring to the decision. Although many decisions taken in the course of the nursery day do not lend themselves easily to making a rational choice – for example, behaviour management, ethical judgements, staffing problems – and are perhaps guided more by time constraints, pressure from parents or a lack of decision-making structure within the team, it is crucial to have a manager with a high level of qualifications and experience. Indeed, many argue that managers should be educated to at least degree level – in order that they have the analytical skills, the ability to think and plan logically, to resist the temptation to let emotional issues cloud the matter.

I would suggest that the skills required of the manager here should relate to the structure of the organisation as a whole. If the manager is unsupported, then she will need such ability at her fingertips; if, however, the manager has support and direction from seniors with whom difficult decisions can be shared, then she is not relying totally on her own knowledge and breadth of experience, but on that of the organisation as a whole.

Routine decisions, which occur frequently, may well have a procedural solution that is well rehearsed in the nursery. Such decisions will not challenge the manager, and will require little discretion or professional judgement. Such a decision is based on previous success, and is sometimes referred to as a 'programmed decision'. All staff should be familiar with the response, and it should be committed to writing in a Procedures Manual (see next section).

Case Study 2

Balancing the needs of children, parents and staff

A rash had broken out in the baby unit. Over the course of two days five babies had developed a rash which, to the manager, looked like measles. However the children were not unwell. Parents were contacted and advised to take their children to their doctors. This produced a variety of diagnoses, none of measles. They ranged from 'miscellaneous viral infection' to 'non-specific allergy' and 'eczema'. None of the GPs was able to confirm that the rash was not contagious.

The parents were keen to return the children to nursery and to return to work themselves, confident with the various doctors' views that the children were not in the first stages of something more serious. However, the staff were concerned that as the outbreak had involved such a significant number of babies then further spread of infection was possible. They made efforts to isolate the children from the older group, just in case. One child in particular began to itch and scratch quite vigorously, although was not upset or considered to be unwell.

Clearly the nursery staff could not deny the advice of the GPs, but the routine in the nursery was being significantly affected by the staff's concern – based on little clear information. Understandably, parents felt there was no real need to exclude the children from nursery. One child had begun to show signs of illness. The local health authority was contacted in order to obtain a view on what action the nursery could take to identify the cause of the rash and therefore the appropriate response. It was not the nursery's role to dispute the diagnosis of a doctor, or to make a judgement on the basis of any one particular doctor's opinion.

A wider problem-solving approach is required for the irregular or new situation that has never been met before. or only infrequently. This may call for a spontaneous reaction, or a considered, customised decision. Such decisions are likely to be made personally by the manager. As we move away from the institutional approach to childcare and education, with increased parental choice and a greater dependence on the private sector – which thrives on diversity – more and more decisions are going to fall into this category. This both acknowledges the importance of comitting the programmed decisions to a Manual, which everyone can follow, and of having a manager capable of rising to the challenge of acquiring decision-making skills in order to cope with a larger number of instances in which such skills will be required.

Carlisle (1979) argued that there are three types of decision (see Case Study 3):

- *intuitive*, i.e. those led by feelings and emotions, regardless of information that might suggest a different response;
- *judgemental*, i.e. those for which the outcome can be predicted because they are based on expert knowledge;
- *problem-solving*, i.e. where time allows study and reflection before a course of action is decided upon.

Intuitive and judgemental decisions are basically taken independently by the leader unless specifically delegated. She is then going to be held accountable for the outcome. The problem-solving approach allows the decision to be shared, and is therefore a less risky strategy, if it can be achieved within the timescale demanded. A manager needs to select the appropriate type of decision-making to ensure that the situation is met with the highest possible quality of decision given the time available. I would add here that indecisiveness or prevarication is rarely an appropriate response where children and parents are involved; however, these are not the same as agreeing to review a policy over time.

In terms of personal risk, decision-making strategies can be ordered as follows (with the most 'risky', i.e. for which the person taking the decision is solely accountable, first):

- individual decision-making by the manager;
- individual decision-making by the acknowledged expert;
- decision-making by averaging the opinions of individuals;
- decision-making by the manager following group discussion;

- decision by a minority;
- decision by a majority;
- decision by consensus.

A good decision is one that is both right and good, and not simply expedient and practical. This is why Codes of Ethics and

---

Case Study 3

Intuitive, judgemental and problem-solving decisions

A vacancy arose for a Senior Nursery Officer and three candidates applied, all from other nurseries within the same network. Two of the candidates had previously worked with the manager at the nursery with the vacancy, who was responsible for interview and selection. The third candidate had worked briefly in the nursery before, providing holiday cover, but at a time when the manager was herself away from the nursery.

The manager's spontaneous reaction to the three candidates was to state a preference for one of the two candidates she had worked with, and to suggest that the one she knew to be outgoing and vivacious would be the most appropriate choice. This was an intuitive decision on the manager's part. Her choice may well have been the right one: she knew her team and who would and would not fit in; she also knew what personal characteristics would contribute something important to the nursery.

However, company procedure stated that all internal candidates must first and foremost be considered in light of recent staff appraisal documentation, and their skills and experience matched to the job specification for the vacancy. This route would result in a judgemental decision – one that can be evidenced and backed up with information.

The judgemental process eliminated one candidate but did not provide a clear choice in favour of either of the remaining candidates. They both met the specification, but in different ways, and personal knowledge of the situations they were intending to vacate added a further dimension. The manager decided to find a solution in conjunction with the two managers of the nurseries they would be leaving, to discuss the pro's and con's from each nursery's point of view. This was a problem-solving approach to finding the right candidate.

Codes of Practice are drawn up for members of professions. Although less developed in the UK than in many other countries, notably Australia and the USA, the Childcare and Education Association in the UK has attempted a Code of Practice to guide private-sector nursery providers. The challenge for nursery managers is to find creative solutions to situations as they arise, which assist the nursery to achieve its task and objectives whilst maintaining harmony amongst the child, parent and staff groups. This requires focus, and developed assertiveness skills.

Planning the Use of Resources

Staffing and everything that goes with it is the most essential and critical aspect of good nursery management. It has already been noted that the quality of service provided relies largely on the quality of the staff. However, to follow through that multi-layered statement, it must be carefully unpacked.

The staff/child ratio

What you say you do must be done. Strangely, this is often not the case. Parents will have been told that you maintain certain staff/child ratios according to the age of the children. Clearly achieving this is not in the application of an exact science, as children change age groups continuously and so the nursery has an amoebic profile, which rarely allows for ratios to be in place, in precise terms. Similarly, children move between different activities and groups in the nursery and frequently groups will exceed the stated ratio because of the popularity of the activity. The staff/child ratio is intended only as a general guide to staffing levels. It allows for child contact and non-contact time and it is highly unlikely that at any given moment the stated staff/child ratios can be precisely observed.

Again, if staff/child ratios are 'always maintained' are they really in place throughout the day? Are all absences of staff truly covered? For example, will all or some of the following give rise to covering staff: lunch breaks, coffee breaks, holidays, staff sickness, training on site and off site, shopping for the nursery, attendance at internal and external meetings, absence of the manager on other business? All these areas leave a gap in the staff/child ratio, either directly or because a member of the team is deputising for the manager.

In addition, if staff are expected to: exchange information with the next shift, undertake child observations, write up child profiles/records, supervise students, be supervised themselves, plan activities, mount artwork, meet with parents, etc., are these routine non-contact tasks absorbed into the (ratio) day? Or are staff given time out and, if so, is it covered by an additional member of staff?

Shift planning

For years my own company worked an 8-hour staff shift, even though our nurseries were open for 10 hours, excluding setting up and closing down time in the mornings and evenings. Because of the need to fit in all those essential absences, as well as the non-contact, on-site tasks, it was impossible to achieve an even spread of staff throughout the day and maintain a viable staff cost. We constantly battled with too few staff in the mornings and evenings, given the workload at those times, and too many staff at times of the day when we needed them least. The only solution was to over-staff, pushing up costs and inevitably increasing fees to parents.

We are currently experimenting with a staff shift of 10 hours, but maintaining a working week of 40 hours; i.e. staff work four days each week instead of five. This allows us to plan staffing accurately against anticipated child attendance. For example, if Friday is less busy in the nursery then staff 'rest days' can be planned to coincide. The 10-hour shift also provides us with a means of achieving high levels of staff from opening to closing time, and in particular has helped with the early and late periods in the day.

There are many issues to take into account when deciding on the right length of shift for your nursery, and you must assess the relative importance of each aspect:

- opening hours;
- patterns of arrival and collection of children;
- parent requirements at both ends of the day;
- variation in daily pattern of occupancy;
- staff contracts of employment;

- commuting patterns of staff;
- incidence of evening meetings;
- extent of non-contact duties;
- use of agency/temporary staff;
- physical separation of nursery rooms.

Staff costs

It is generally considered that, to achieve a high quality of service, salary costs (including agency fees or temporary staff wages) should not be less than 50% of the nursery's turnover – i.e. fees received from or on behalf of parents. Without doubt, staff costs are the element of total costs that it is crucial to control: measure the effect on the economics of the nursery of a 5% overspend on salary costs, against a 5% variance on any other item. It is therefore entirely appropriate for staffing requirements to be driven by total fees (or equivalent) expected. Careful control of forward bookings in the nursery, and actual child attendance, are together the most prudent route for planning staff resources (Figure 2).

Policies and Procedures

Why do we need to specify our policies and why do we need written procedures? Surely these things deny professional judgement and preclude imaginative response.

Providing consistency for children and parents, and empowering staff to be flexible, is not a contradiction in terms. The first allows the second to be approached with confidence and with the full support of the team.

The smooth running of the nursery relies on routines being respected and achieved. There are many safeguards to put in place, particularly stemming from health and safety regulations, equal opportunities practice, child protection measures, local authority registration requirements and, last but not least, the contract for services made with parents. It is an absolute entitlement of children and parents that they can rely on all these requirements being in place, every minute of every day. My purpose here is not to rehearse such standard and basic elements of a nursery service, but to look beyond entitlements of children, to better practice.

	Mon a.m.	Mon p.m.	Tue a.m.	Tue p.m.	Wed a.m.	Wed p.m.	Thu a.m.	Thu p.m.	Fri a.m.	Fri p.m.
Total under-2s × 5 booked hrs	17	17	18	18	19	19	17	17	16	16
U2 total hrs U2 ratio 1:3	85.0	85.0	90.0	90.0	95.0	95.0	85.0	85.0	80.0	80.0
Staff hours	28.3	28.3	30.0	30.0	31.7	31.7	28.3	28.3	26.7	26.7
Total 2–3s × 5 booked hrs	11	11	14	14	16	16	16	16	15	15
2–3 total hrs 2–3 ratio 1:4	55.0	55.0	70.0	70.0	80.0	80.0	80.0	80.0	75.0	75.0
Staff hours	13.8	13.8	17.5	17.5	20.0	20.0	20.0	20.0	18.8	18.8
Total 3–5s × 5 booked hrs	5	5	5	5	5	5	4	4	3	3
3–5 total hrs 3–5 ratio 1:8	25.0	25.0	25.0	25.0	25.0	25.0	20.0	20.0	15.0	15.0
Staff hours	3.1	3.1	3.1	3.1	3.1	3.1	2.5	2.5	1.9	1.9
Total staff hours	45.2	45.2	50.6	50.6	54.8	54.8	50.8	50.8	47.4	47.4
Staff required	**9.0**	**9.0**	**10.1**	**10.1**	**11.0**	**11.0**	**10.2**	**10.2**	**9.5**	**9.5**

	Mon	Tue	Wed	Thu	Fri
Carol	1	1	RD	1	1
Mary	RD	1	1	AL	1
Alex	RD	1	1	1	1
Fiona	RD	1	1	1	1
Lorraine	1	1	1	1	RD
Karen	1	RD	1	1	1
Julie	1	1	RD	1	1
Claire	1	1	1	1	RD
Susan	1	RD	1	1	1
Tracy	1	1	1	RD	1
Joe	1	RD	1	1	1
Lynda	1	1	1	RD	1
Permanent staff	9	9	10	9	10
Agency	0	1	1	1	0
Jennifer (Manager)	1	1	1	1	1
Staff on site	**10**	**11**	**12**	**11**	**11**

Figure 2. An example of staff planning for one week (AL = annual leave, RD = rest day).

Written procedures reduce the incidence of misunderstanding as to the standard of the measure put in place. They allow parents and staff to predict how matters will be dealt with. They provide a basis for review and improvement of procedures. And they do not leave the nursery vulnerable when the person who 'knows about that' is absent (see Case Study 4).

Written procedures reflect state-of-the-art childcare, and as such are your defence if questioned on the standard of services you

---

Case Study 4

A written policy would help

It was the end of February and everyone who hadn't had a cold all winter now had one. The sun had not shone for months and many children were left with lingering coughs and catarrh. They needed extra help settling for naps and kept each other awake. This was getting to be a strain for everyone, and parents were frustrated at collecting irritable children at the end of the day and going through the whole process again at bedtime. Calpol helped at home, and so it was suggested by a parent that a spoonful would also aid the midday nap. This particular child had been very susceptible to the colds going round and had had more than the average time away from nursery because of this.

The nursery had a clear written policy about the administration of prescribed drugs in nursery. It also had a clear written policy that, in the incidence of an abnormal temperature, Calpol would be given having sought the parent's specific permission, in the intervening period between telephoning the parent and the child being collected. There was no written policy about the administration of non-prescribed drugs in any other circumstances.

The parent wanted the nursery to administer Calpol to aid sleep whilst the child's cough continued. The nursery refused. The parent sought advice from the local authority, who considered that where a parent's permission had been specifically requested and received, then the nursery could do this. The member of staff had no written policy to support her view that it was inappropriate for the nursery to administer over-the-counter medicines except where the child was unwell. Had she had this, a heated discussion in the nursery could have been avoided as it would not have been an issue for negotiation.

offer. It is important that you can rely on the fact that *all* your staff will deal with a particular issue in the same way, thus providing consistency of service. You can be even more certain that this will happen if staff understand *why* procedures have developed. What is the objective of having a procedure for that particular nursery function or routine?

External Pressure for Written Policies

As part of the government's nursery voucher scheme, which is due to be implemented nationwide in April 1997, nurseries wishing to redeem vouchers are required to publish comprehensive information about their policies and procedures. The documents published by the Department for Education and Employment (DFEE 1996) envisage that such information will include:

- staffing policy, including number of staff, their qualifications and training;
- educational programmes and activity;
- record-keeping, progress recording, reporting to parents;
- premises and equipment available;
- health and safety policies;
- equal opportunity policies;
- special educational needs policy and how it is implemented;
- admission policy;
- opening hours, dates and daily programme;
- discipline policy;
- fees;
- complaints procedure;
- copy of the last Children Act or OFSTED report.

The information must be made available so that parents are given 'plenty of time to reach their decision'.

As a condition of initial registration for the receipt of vouchers, providers will be required to publish information, including, but by no means restricted to, a statement of the education that will be provided. The published statement will provide the framework for planning which can demonstrate that it builds on children's experience and achievement, and responds to individual needs. Confirmation of eligibility for voucher status will be based on a judgement, through inspection, about the extent to which the quality of the provision is appropriate to the Schools Curriculum Assessent Authority's (SCAA) desirable learning outcomes, rather than on the achievement of the outcomes themselves by individual children.

The government's voucher scheme will then require all nurseries wishing to participate to commit to writing what they do and to demonstrate how they do it.

A Manual of Policies and Procedures

Written procedures are best produced as reference manuals that can be readily updated. The more well-thumbed the manual, the more consistent your service is likely to be. The more familiar staff are with the manual, the more likely it is that they will contribute to its review and updating. Like any manual, it will evolve over time and be a living, learning information resource. It may begin with the fulfilment of the nursery's registration criteria, which will cover the essential areas noted earlier, of health and safety, equal opportunities, special educational needs, and child protection.

The manual should then expand to incorporate areas of good practice that are not regulated under the Children Act, and further, to include aspects of quality provision consistent with your nursery's commitment to children and parents (Figure 3). It is important that each procedure carries any relevant cross-references to other procedures, and that the manual is kept up to date with current information, such as names, addresses, etc.

Each policy or procedure should begin with a statement of what the objective is – i.e. for what purpose a policy or a procedure is being laid down, and for whose benefit there should be a standardised way of handling the issue.

Philosophy

There should be an overall statement of the nursery's intention and approach to childcare. It can include references to the underlying principles of early learning to which the nursery relates (e.g. Montessori, Froebel, Piaget, a blend . . .) and it can explain how parents might detect that these principles are at work in the nursery.

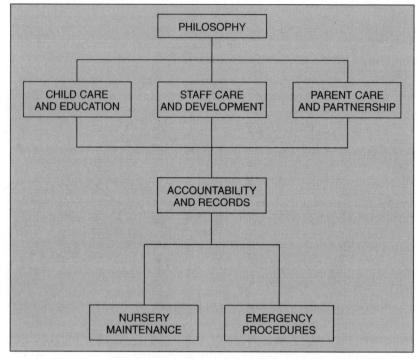

Figure 3.   A framework for a manual that incorporates all standard procedures carried out in a nursery.

Child care and education

This section should cover all the childcare routines and activities that are required to be undertaken in accordance with an agreed policy. Each procedure should clearly indicate the minimum legal requirements as provided for within the nursery's registration if such a requirement is made, and the nursery's own (higher) standard, if relevant. A typical contents list in this section would cover:

- Admission Policy
- Settling Children into the Nursery
- Staff Ratios and Qualifications
- Keyworking System
- Early Years' Curriculum
- Activity Planning and Evaluation
- Mounting and Display of Artwork

- Observation of Children's Profiles
- Service Quality Observation
- Child Discipline
- Meals
- Multi-Cultural Images
- Gender Policy
- Children with Special Needs
- Hygiene
- Health and Safety
- First Aid
- HIV and Hepatitis B
- Non-accidental injury (NAI)
- Child Protection
- Sick Children
- Children's Outings
- Collection of Children from the Nursery
- Relationship with Statutory Authorities and Local Community
- Relationship with Wider Community
- Visitors to the Nursery

An example of one of these procedures is given in Figure 4.

Staff care and development

The section on staff care would cover the following areas:

- Terms and Conditions of Employment
- Equal Opportunities
- Staff Recruitment Procedures
- Induction Training
- Training and Development
- Supervision
- Staff Appraisal
- Disciplinary Procedures
- Grievance Procedures
- Domestic/Maintenance Staff
- Students
- Volunteers

An example of one of these procedures is given in Figure 5. A sample staff appraisal form is included as an appendix to this chapter.

MOUNTING AND DISPLAY OF ARTWORK

OBJECTIVE

To ensure display tables and mounted artwork are always presented attractively so that the children's work is the focal point.

PROCEDURE

When mounting artwork the display area should be defined by first backing the pinboard to highlight the area being used to display. Each individual piece of work should be backed at least once and when put up it should be symmetrical and in-line. Artwork should not be displayed at angles unless this enhances a project.

Backing paper should always be in unobtrusive colours so that the focus is on the child's piece of work.

A child's picture should never be cut after completion and paper should never be pre-shaped in order to influence the child's creativity. The only exception however would be, for example, a shape project that was enhanced by the use of shaped paper. This method should be used cautiously.

Names should always be clearly printed in the left-hand corner so that the child understands the convention is left-to-right. Only the initial letter should be in capitals. If a child does not want his or her name on a piece of work the issue should not be forced and a compromise sought; i.e. 'Can I put your name on the back so as not to spoil your picture, then we will know it is yours?'

Handwriting should always be of a high standard and there should be no compromises on this issue. If there are good neat handwriters within the team others should be encouraged to use them. The company has a set of guidelines for letter formation which should be followed carefully. Each nursery agrees a universal alphabet so that each handwriter uses the same formation. Rulers should never be used by staff to keep print straight as they produce flat-bottomed letters.

Artwork should be replaced and refreshed regularly, and staples, BlueTack etc. should always be removed immediately. PrittStick and staples must not be used on walls. Unobtrusive methods of fixing should be used where possible; e.g. dress-making pins with a pin pusher.

Where appropriate, paper should be recycled (e.g. backing paper used more than once) for children's work.

Staples should be applied at an angle to ensure easy removal.

Paper should always be cut straight and a guillotine used to do this.

Figure 4. Example of a child care and education procedure.

Parent care and partnership

The parent care section should cover:

- Partnership with Parents
- Parent Enquiries

STAFF APPRAISAL

OBJECTIVE

To ensure that staff receive regular and constructive feedback on their progress and that they have the opportunity to discuss privately any aspect of work or relationships that concerns them.

To redefine the professional development needs of the individual and to set out a programme for its fulfilment.

PROCEDURE

Staff are appraised at the end of their probationary period and then on a six-monthly basis in October and April.

The appraisal discussion takes place in private between the coordinator and member of staff and is based on the sections and headings of the appraisal form.

Staff are notified at least five working days in advance of the date and time of their appraisal meeting and are given a copy of the appraisal form at that time to enable them to prepare for the meeting.

At the end of the appraisal meeting the appraisee is invited to enter any comments in the appropriate section of the form and to sign it.

All staff are entitled to have a copy of their appraisal if they so wish.

Figure 5.   Example of a staff care and development procedure.

- Showing Parents Around the Nursery
- Parent Contract
- Parent Contact/Meetings
- Consultation Group

An example of one of these procedures is given in Figure 6.

Accountability and records

The accountability section covers all areas of reporting for which the nursery manager is responsible. In some cases this will be information requested by the owner/company, and in others it will be prepared for the purposes of the Management Group/Committee to which the manager reports. Certain reports are required by law, as provided for in the Children Act, and will be subject to inspection by the local authority. These are Incident, Accident and Complaints reports, together with the Register of children.

CONSULTATION GROUP

PURPOSE

The Consultation Group acts as a consultative body primarily to make recommendations for the further enhancement of the nursery services. The Group monitors standards, facilities and services provided, to ensure that they continue to be relevant to the needs of clients and in line with good practice.

MEMBERSHIP

The Group includes nursery management, parents, employer representatives and relevant local individuals who can bring influence and contribute to the continuous development of the nursery. The Group will include:

- Company Managing Director
- Company Operations Manager
- Nursery Coordinator
- One representative from each participating employer
- Two parent representatives.

It is desirable that the Group also includes:

- Nursery Deputy Coordinator
- One nominated local primary headteacher
- One representative from the local NNEB training college
- One represenative from the participating developer, where relevant.

TERMS OF REFERENCE

The Group will receive:

- A Nursery Coordinator's report, covering numbers of children, staff changes, and information on special projects/developments and staff training.
- A parent representatives' report, covering any issues received by the parent representatives that require discussion on nursery policy, i.e. those issues that cannot be resolved through the day-to-day practice of parent/nursery partnership.
- Items for discussion raised by the company representatives.

The above standard agenda items are intended to set the scene for ideas and discussion with respect to the ongoing development of the service provided by the nursery. The nursery management is also responsible for bringing to the notice of the Group any issues that may warrant discussion in the Group; these may include changes in legislation/public policy or company policy.

OPERATION

The Consultation Group will meet every three months, i.e. four meetings each year. At least two weeks' notice should be given of meetings, which will normally be held at the nursery.

An Agenda will be drawn up by the Nursery Coordinator who will contact both parent and company representatives beforehand. The meetings will normally be chaired by the Coordinator, and will be minuted. Minutes will be posted on the Nursery Parents' Noticeboard and distributed to all members of the Group.

Figure 6. Example of a parent care and partnership procedure.

Other matters are orderly accounting and record-keeping, and form part of the properly run nursery's quality assurance package (see Chapter 7). The accountability section is likely to cover the following:

- Accountability
- Children's Applications
- Children's Records
- Staff Records
- Local Purchases and Local Repairs
- Financial Administration
- Nursery Income/Expenditure Reporting
- Incident Reports
- Accident Reports
- Enquiries and Nursery Bookings Reporting
- Staff Planning
- Shift/Rota Planning
- Complaints
- Correspondence
- Filing

An example of one of these procedures is given in Figure 7.

INCIDENT REPORTS

OBJECTIVE

To establish an accurate record of any incident that occurs at the nursery or to any member of staff or child in nursery operating time which may need to be recounted at a later date.

PROCEDURE

On being informed of an incident that needs to be recorded, the Coordinator should immediately gain as much information as possible. The incident form should be completed immediately.

The Coordinator should then use his/her discretion about reporting the incident immediately to Head Office. This should be done for any event requiring communication to any external body/individual.

At all times the parents/carers should be informed of any incident and a copy of the form offered to them.

Figure 7.   Example of an accountability procedure.

Nursery maintenance

The Rumbold report (1990) said that 'Educators and their architects need to ensure that the learning environment both inside and out is well designed and organised so as to be accessible, comprehensible and stimulating for the children; that equipment is appropriate and in satisfactory condition; and that the best use is made of the particular opportunities offered by the locality.' It is equally important to ensure that the nursery layout facilitates supervision of children, and is flexible to the changing day-by-day space needs. Children and staff need to feel secure in their environment, and staff do not want to use precious time on 'policing' different corners of the nursery, rather than interacting with children in a focused and undistracted way. Equally children and staff like to redefine their space, to suit the needs of the group utilising the particular area of the nursery, to create a fresh arrangement, to juxtapose activity areas in better ways.

The nursery environment is critical to the performance of the service and this section of the manual will reflect your concern with that aspect.

Clearly the relationship between the nurture of positive attitudes towards the nursery environment and health and safety is close. But it is also about making life easier for staff, so that they can concentrate on what they are uniquely capable of doing, and developing children's attitudes towards space, property, and respect for what other people are doing. The contents list in this section may cover:

- Nursery Design and Layout
- Opening and Closing Procedures
- Cleaning
- Equipment Servicing
- Building Repairs and Equipment Repair/Replacement
- Housekeeping Standards
- Fire Drill
- Crime Prevention

An example of one of these procedures is given in Figure 8.

Emergency procedures

This is the last, but by no means least important, section of any

CLEANING

OBJECTIVE

To ensure that the nursery is maintained to the highest standards of cleanliness and hygiene.

PROCEDURES

The general cleaning of the nursery should take place out of operating hours, either in the early morning or after the nursery closes at night. Daily cleaning must include the following:

- sweeping of external paths and patio areas
- cleaning/vacuuming of entrance lobby
- mopping of floor
- dusting of display surfaces and ledges and cleaning of work/play surfaces
- thorough cleaning of toilets, wash basins, mirrors and of kitchen equipment and surfaces.

Windows should be cleaned monthly though it may be necessary for some windows to be cleaned more frequently.

It is the responsibility of nursery staff during the day to ensure that the nursery is constantly maintained in a clean and hygienic condition. Accidents and spills must be attended to immediately and the kitchen and other food areas should be thoroughly cleaned after food preparation and meals.

Figure 8. Example of a nursery maintenance procedure.

nursery manual. The procedures here need to be unequivocally clear and cover all possible eventualities. By their very nature, they will need to be read, absorbed, rehearsed and acted upon quickly and smoothly. They also combine the absolute minimum in terms of procedures that each and every individual member of staff, however temporary, should be aware of.

Clearly in this section it is *vital* to maintain current telephone numbers, nominated individuals, authorities, etc.

Certain emergency procedures should be displayed, usually as bullet-point instructions, as well as comprising part of the reference manual. They are basic health and safety precautions and will be required to be in place not only as part of the nursery registration, but also as an essential prerequisite of insurance policies relating to children, staff, visitors and premises. The contents in this section of the manual should cover as a minimum:

- Fire
- Break-in

FIRE EMERGENCY PROCEDURE

If you discover fire (and cannot put it out at once), raise the alarm immediately.

The Coordinator/Deputy is responsible for telephoning the fire brigade and Head Office. In their absence the most senior on duty has the responsibility.

The Coordinator or Deputy should check that the building is empty of children, staff and other visitors. Close the doors and windows, if it is safe to do so, and then leave the building by the nearest exit. If it has not yet been collected, they should take the attendance form as they leave.

In the event of a fire breaking out in the kitchen, the cook should if possible turn off electrical and gas appliances before leaving.

Once outside, all occupants of the nursery should go straight to the assembly point under the chestnut tree in front of the office building. The Coordinator/Deputy will then use the attendance form to check that everyone is safe.

Figure 9.   Example of an emergency procedure.

- Theft
- Power Cut
- Bomb Scare
- Accident
- Illness
- Failure to Collect a Child

An example of one of these procedures is given in Figure 9.

Appendices

The comprehensive nursery manual will have a number of appendices. These may include reference points, such as a copy of the registration document, the National Children's Bureau's *Guidelines for Good Practice*, the Schools Curriculum Assessment Authority's *Desirable Learning Outcomes*, and your own full set of brochure material. It may also include a pack of standard letters/documentation used with parents and with staff. It can also include a full set of sample children's records documentation. Anything not included, but used in a standard format, should be clearly referenced as part of expected practice and daily use.

Appendix to Chapter 2

Appraisal Form: Nursery Officer

Name..

Position ....

Date of appointment ....

Date of appraisal ....

Introduction to the Appraisal Form

1. The purpose of this form is to assist the appraiser and appraisee reach agreement in evaluating job performance and then determining what further help or training is needed for career development.

2. The form is in four parts:

    PART ONE   Measures performance in relation to the agreed responsibilities and accountabilities set out in the job description.

    PART TWO   Measures performance in relation to the personal qualities or skills that are agreed to be most appropriate to the requirements of the job.

    PART THREE   Provides space for the appraiser to record the action or further assistance needed to enable the appraisee to improve job performance and achieve career progression.

    PART FOUR   Provides space for the appraisee to enter any comments that he or she wishes to make.

3. In PARTS ONE and TWO, the appraiser and apraisee need to agree a performance rating for the responsibility, personal quality or skill under discussion. The scale is as follows:

    5   Excellent quality
    4   Very good
    3   Expected competency
    2   Poor – considerable scope for improvement
    1   Very weak – major improvement required urgently

    Entries in PART ONE (reproduced here) relate to the job being performed and not necessarily to the person carrying out the job. For example, if the appraisee is new to the position, the rating will not necessarily reflect the contribution of the appraisee. However, if the appraisee has held the position for a long time, the ratings will reflect on the person and the job.

4. In all cases the appraisee should receive a copy of this form at least one week before the appraisal meeting and be asked to complete PARTS ONE and TWO in readiness for the discussion.

    The appraiser will also complete PARTS ONE and TWO.

    The meeting itself will then seek consensus on the performance ratings and the action and assistance needed.

    PART FOUR is for the appraisee to enter any comments on the appraisal.

PART ONE: RESPONSIBILITIES AND ACCOUNTABILITIES

Enter below the appraisee's key responsibilities from the job description.

KEY RESPONSIBILITIES	RATING
1. *To ensure that the children are cared for in a happy stimulating environment following the principles of childcare embodied in the company's Nursery Manual.*	
• familiarity, acceptance and demonstrations of expectations and philosophies stated in the manual	
• contribution to the creation and maintenance of a stimulating and challenging environment for the children	
• ability to make appropriate and efficient use of teaching space	
• ability to devise relevant and interesting activities and experiences	
• ability to use stimulating resources	
• ability to plan a suitable range and balance of activity	
• consistency of mood-friendliness, warmth and good nature at all times	
2. *To ensure that the developmental needs of children are met within a framework of planned activity that also enables learning to take place within an anti-racist and non-sexist environment.*	
• provision of activities to match current learning needs of children	
• ability to respond appropriately to the initiatives demonstrated by the children	
• awareness of the potential learning opportunities embodied within the range of activities	
• ability to focus children's attention and maximise upon learning opportunities	
• ability to modify teaching in the light of individual responses	
• ability to make the most of young children's curiosity	
• awareness of the need to encourage equal opportunities, e.g. boys in the home corner, girls in the bricks	
• demonstration that all children and cultures are valued as common practice	
• to maximise opportunities to promote the positive benefits of living in a pluralistic society	
• provision of opportunities for first-hand experimentation, exploration, observation, discussion and investigation	
NOTES:	

KEY RESPONSIBILITIES	RATING
3. *To ensure that high standards of hygiene and safety are maintained at all times and that the policies and procedures of the nursery are correctly followed.*	
• establishment of good working relationships with the children	
• calmness and manner of dealing with difficult situations/behaviour	
• ability to redirect children when necessary	
• ability to organise and direct the children	
• ability safely to organise and maintain materials and equipment in both short and long term	
• ability to anticipate potentially unsafe or disruptive situations and divert	
• compliance with expected health and safety routines, e.g. hand-washing, kitchen vigilance, first aid, fire drills, general safety awareness	
• ability to exude a sense of security by having clear expectations and defining boundaries to children	
• being supportive of other staff and presenting a united approach	
• ability to ensure that activities taking place at the same time are compatible	
• ability to manage own activity while keeping an overview of the rest of the activities in the nursery	
• awareness of other children in the nursery when engaged with own group	
4. *To keep careful observations of the children within the keyworker role, building up a full profile of each through close liaison with other agencies, supporting staff concerned with each child, and meaningful and regular dialogue with parents or carers.*	
• ability to form effective warm relationships with children	
• willingness and ability to make contact with parents	
• openness to creating links with other agencies	
• initiating and maintaining dialogue with other staff members	
• ability to talk knowledgeably about given children	
• ability to keep meaningful notes	
• ability to observe children and recognise what is meaningful to them	
• ability to intervene appropriately in children's activities	
• ability to make an assessment of each child's needs	
• assessing quality of the relationship with parents and recognising when there is strain	
NOTES:	

KEY RESPONSIBILITIES	RATING
5. *To cooperate and communicate with the Coordinator and Deputy on all nursery matters, contribute to staff meetings, participate as a responsible member of the team, and present a professional code of conduct at all times.*	
• appearance – attitude – speech	
• punctuality	
• reliability	
• vitality	
• sensitivity to situations	
• ability to identify own strengths and weaknesses and complement other team members/training	
• willingness to ask for and act upon advice	
• willingness to develop a rapport and good professional relationships with staff	
• contribute to staff meetings/participate as a responsible member of the team and any other occasions when representing the company	
• willingness to attend conferences/meetings etc.	
NOTES:	

COMMENTS FROM APPRAISER
PERFORMANCE:
CAREER DEVELOPMENT PLAN:
Signed ....(appraisee) Date ....

3

Leading a Team and Managing a Service

- Motivation and Commitment
- Roles and Responsibilities
- Teamwork
- The Team Manager
- Dealing with Conflicts
- Selling the Nursery
- Working to a Plan
- Furthering the Quality of Service
- Planning Staff Shifts
- Communication
- Personal Well-being
- Managing Yourself and Others
- Conclusion
- Appendix

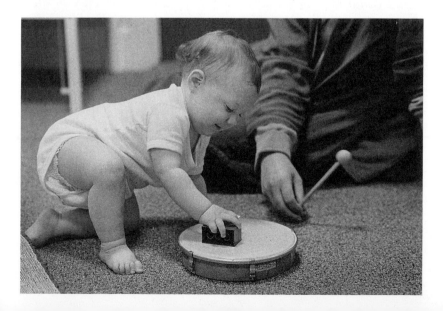

Motivation and Commitment

There has been much written about the personal and professional attributes of those providing non-parental care and education of young children, which has drawn a great deal of public attention, particularly in the residential care sector. Researchers in the pre-school field have consistently drawn attention to the low status or reward predicament of nursery nurses and teachers. Whitebuck *et al.* (1989) and others highlighted the influence of staff disaffection and turnover on children's social and language development; Penn (1994) identified direct links between parent satisfaction with ser-vices, and conditions of employment. Guidance to the Children Act issued by the Department of Health recognises this research to the extent that it draws attention to the rights of people working with young children. Similarly, Angela Rumbold (1990) said that:

> 'The status afforded to any group or profession has an impor-tant influence on the recognition and support it secures for itself. Yet adults working with under fives have traditionally enjoyed less esteem than those working with children of statu-tory school age, outside and even within the ranks of the pro-fessions themselves. This is reflected in substantial measure, in terms of pay, moreover differences of relative status between groups concerned with the under fives go beyond those inherent in, or flowing or receiving from, their different level of training. Besides coming within different sets of arrangements for pay and conditions of service, the groups differ markedly in their opportunities for in-service training – though all alike suffer limitations in their career prospects.'

It is noteworthy that one of the imperatives that has been a driv-ing force behind the establishment of many independent sector nurseries is the need for employers to retain staff. Yet how effec-tive are we at this very aspect of management? Not very effective, according to Penn.

A nursery manager needs to be aware of the components that each of the various training routes for work with under-fives should deliver. Figure 10 shows that alongside the formal and tra-ditional training route, there is also the system of accreditation introduced in 1991, embedded in National Vocational

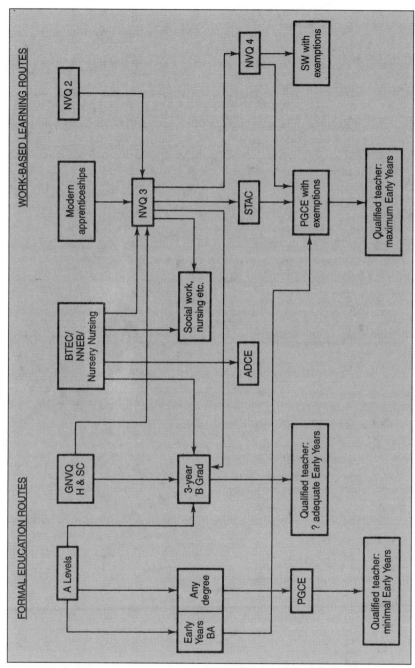

Figure 10.   Emerging models of training for early years' workers.

Qualifications (NVQs). NVQs are competency-based qualifications, as distinct from knowledge-based, which is what had gone before. Candidates are assessed in the workplace, and links have been established to equate NVQ competency levels with traditional qualifications.

At the time of writing, it is sad to have to note that despite the links being made, and NVQ competencies being accepted as both relevant and equivalent in terms of the actual skills and abilities of under-fives staff, many local authorities do not recognise this training route and will not consider staff as 'qualified'. The jury is then still out on whether NVQs have brought about a rise in status for people working with under-fives.

One of the few aspects of early years' service provision that all commentators seem to agree on is that quality of service, in large measure, depends on continuity in the staff team. How can we attract good staff in the first place and encourage commitment?

I recently conducted a small survey amongst industry colleagues, of the terms and conditions which they felt reflected the priorities of incoming staff. In order of priority the list ran:

1. salary
2. holiday allowance
3. sick pay
4. other financial benefits: clothing allowance, pension, maternity pay, childcare subsidy
5. nursery philosophy
6. roles and responsibilities
7. nursery premises and equipment
8. career development opportunities.

Putting the same question to the test on my own staff, I found that priorities differed:

1. nursery philosophy
2. nursery premises and equipment
3. in-service training
4. career development opportunities
5. holiday allowance
6. salary
7. other financial benefits.

The point to be made here is that a nursery manager should

understand what it is about the setting that staff find attractive, and try to identify what can be provided over time to encourage staff to stay.

I was pleasantly surprised to learn that, far from being overly-competitive about benefits packages in the City of London, there is a network of Human Resource Managers who exchange information and share new ideas about staff retention, in order that as a whole they are supporting a constant stream of good applicants into the sector. One of the purposes of the Childcare and Education Association, a professional body for private-sector childcare providers, is to exchange information and experiences for the benefit of the industry as a whole. However, as yet, this has not extended to staff remuneration packages.

But, although every nursery hopes to keep its good people, it must also survive financially. It is not possible simply to go on paying people more money for doing the same job, even though they may be doing it better or more efficiently and bringing more experience to bear. The nursery manager has to employ more subtle means than pay, to sustain commitment. My own staff's priority list suggests that, in any event, salary is not the only or even the most highly-rated reward that nursery staff seek.

The importance of understanding, sharing in and contributing to nursery philosophy is dealt with in Chapter 5. Suffice it to say here, that belonging to 'a team' and making a long-term commitment means being able to sign up to the team's objectives, working with – not despite – the flow. It relates to inclusion (Chapter 1) and being involved in change (Chapter 7).

It is reasonable that nursery staff should expect to work in an environment that allows them to practise the skills and knowledge they have acquired. Skills and knowledge will go on developing, but without an equivalent development in the way space is arranged, or material resources received and obtained, staff will be limited in their ability to put their plans into action. Without doubt this will lead to professional frustration.

The emphasis that is placed on training and continuous professional development underlines the recognition that childcare is not a service that stands still in terms of what staff need to know. In relative terms, I have not been in the provision of nurseries as a business endeavour for very long, a mere 6 years. However, in that time the goalposts of recognised quality have been dramatically and forcefully moved several times. In 1989 the Children Act brought with it new and higher minimum standards; their predecessors had held good for 50-odd years! Media interest in childcare since has heightened the awareness of parents and encouraged them to be discriminating in their choice; the intended government childcare voucher scheme has imposed the achievement of 'learning outcomes' on pre-school settings. All these initiatives constitute new yardsticks, new standards that quickly become the base entitlement of children and the basic expectation of parents. Such standards draw on, but do no necessarily entirely adopt, contemporary research and thinking into the way children develop and learn. But if we accept the research and the thinking, shouldn't that *higher* target become our goal?

So, qualifications provide the gateposts to a career. But traditional skills need updating, and new knowledge needs to be acquired. My own company requires a commitment to training from every member of staff. My responsibility is then to identify what is needed related to the service we offer, and to provide it. As we know, nursery nursing has suffered from having a low ceiling in career terms. Many career moves that are made are sideways, rather than up, and are made for the reasons of improved conditions rather than increased responsibility. So experience is broadened, but not even this is necessarily recognised in terms of status or reward.

The private sector is beginning to sort itself out. We have, on the whole, moved out of the embryonic phase of development, where the industry was made up of individuals attempting to do all these things for staff within the context of operating one nursery project. There are now a number of post-recession survivors who are beginning to cooperate on a number of different levels: locally as an information network; through Early Years' Forums, across local authority areas to exchange experiences; through associations; forming partnerships; merging.

This will increase the scope for planned career developments on the part of employers, as they will be able to provide opportunities across more than one site, and retain their investment in people.

Roles and Responsibilities

A nursery is not like an office. Whereas office workers can settle in each morning, with a coffee or a chat, or even get stuck straight into writing, making telephone calls or a business meeting, it is not an option for nursery staff to put people off until they feel ready for the conversation. Children and parents rely on the nursery to have a routine, which is not adjustable to suit staff preferences or personal priorities. Upholding a routine requires each and every individual staff team member to know what is expected of them at all points in the day: what and who they are responsible for; where they are based in the nursery; and which tasks are to be completed. If there is any room for misunderstanding in any aspects of this, then child, parent and colleague are let down.

But a nursery team is not a regiment, and neither should a good nursery feel like an institution. The planning and processes that allow the nursery to function smoothly should not be allowed to overpower the objective of offering the blend of warmth and professionalism that we all seek.

Goldschmied and Jackson (1994) warn us against the takeover of 'institutional rush'. This is where the important aspect or phase of an activity or period in a day is overwhelmed by the need to prepare for the next activity or period. Goldschmied and Jackson cite the example of a lunchtime they observed, where there was a harmful and disturbing sense that the meal had to be got over with. This was traced to the fact that the staff who washed up had a contract which meant they had to finish by 1 p.m. This deadline had a ripple effect back to the moment when the children sat down at their tables. How much social interaction was lost, and how much sheer pleasure in the meal was forgone by children and staff?

For a manager, defining roles and responsibilities focuses on the following challenges:

- How can we ensure that 'institutional rush' does not take over?
- How can we ensure that the nursery runs smoothly, and that there is time for play and rest?
- How can we ensure that one activity runs smoothly into another, to reduce the incidence of children roaming in an unfocused way?
- How can we ensure that each member of the team knows how to bring the best out in each other and understands the importance of teamwork?

There is a hierarchy of traditional personnel tools available to promote understanding of individual responsibilities, and of how these fit into the overall scheme for roles within an organisation. They form the building blocks for staff to know whether or not they are getting their roles right. The most important components are the job description, the induction programme, and staff appraisal (see the appendix to Chapter 2). These standard components should be drawn up, having considered the breakdown of responsibilities which need to be covered by nursery staff (see Figure 11).

Many of the areas of responsibility listed in Figure 11 are dealt with in some detail in other chapters of the book. Here I would like to focus on those important management issues that arise over and over again in daily practice, and principally relate to people working well, or not so well, together.

You might say that the list of responsibilities may equally apply to a good nursery nurse as to a nursery manager, particularly as far as the first three categories in Figure 11 are concerned. However, the comment would not be inconsistent with the central theme of this book that managerial responsibility should be totally integrated into the professional role. When accepting the job as manager, you do not go through a metamorphosis and leave behind you everything you know and the way you approach your core discipline of nursery nursing or teaching. On the contrary, you have been selected because of your abilities in these areas, to develop your experience of managing others in those more specialist roles.

The functions of leadership, over and above the management role, were discussed in Chapter 2. It was noted that leadership is frequently shared across a number of (and sometimes all) staff in a nursery. This has a lot to do with *empowerment* – providing staff with the skills and authority to take decisions and respond to the needs of the situation as they arise. It is why many nursery managers are not called 'Manager' or 'Director', but rather 'Coordinator' or 'Head of Centre' – terms that imply the existence of a team.

Teamwork

Nursery services involve a number of sets of people, their relationships, and their feelings. Managing these relies on the subor-

Children-related responsibilities:

* programme of activities
* care routines
* maintaining occupancy

Staff-related responsibilities:

* recruitment and employment
* support and direction
* deployment and teamwork
* development and training

Parent-related responsibilities:

* liaison and contracts
* participation and partnership
* feedback

Organisation-related responsibilities:

* finance
* administration
* marketing

Outside responsibilities:

* registration and inspection
* liaison with related professions, e.g. health, education
* local community

Figure 11. Breakdown of responsibilities.

dination of individual interests and needs in order jointly to provide coordinated activities to achieve common purposes. This is why teamwork is important.

No nursery would wish to think that it has anything but an open and welcoming atmosphere. Achieving this has much to do with the outlook of staff and fulfilment in their posts. *The basic requirements for working well together are*:

* shared aims and objectives;
* a common working language;
* the ability to manage relationships as well as tasks.

Setting out the aims and objectives of the nursery as a whole is discussed in Chapter 6 in some detail. In order that each individual can feel valued and take personal responsibility for the quality of their contribution, they must know where and for what, together and jointly, the staff team is aiming. To exclude a team member from acquiring this is both demeaning and demoralising, and undermines the knowledge and experience they bring with them to their job.

In discussion of aims and objectives, it is equally important that no member of the team feels excluded because of the principles on which the aims and objectives are based. I am referring here to basic assumptions and attitudes towards children and parents, equal opportunities and work. In our nurseries, our vocabulary does not include 'kids', 'naughty', 'bad'; we do not sit in judgement over parents who work long days, or staff who need to respect cultural patterns that prevent them from joining in social events. The ground rules need to be established in order that each and every member feels secure, as if they belong. The manager's role is to set out the ground rules to identify when they need developing and to act as a role model in making them work. These ideas are further expanded in Chapter 7.

As a member of a team, you will have certain responsibilities assigned to you which will involve a number of tasks to be accomplished. As a manager, many of your tasks will be to ensure that others fulfil their responsibilities appropriately. Ensuring that somebody does something involves not only making sure that the task is understood, but that the individual is willing and able to undertake it. The manager is then concerned with the relationship of one member of staff to another, and how the delegation of tasks and deployment of staff affects them as people. An individual may be the right person to do something, but someone else may be making it difficult in some way for that task to be carried out. The manager needs to unblock this situation.

Teamwork recognises a current belief in the value of *management by participation* – working together as equal members of a team provides social support that relieves the strain and stress of nursery life. Group morale can be influenced for better or worse by the disposition of any one member.

But the 'team leader', the nursery manager, is still held responsible for the achievements and failures of a team. The nursery manager is responsible for taking the team from birth to maturity (Rodd 1994).

Getting together

The first stage of the development of a team is when a group of people become aware that they are going to be working together. The clock in Figure 12 illustrates the ensuing phases in the development. Even though a team may feel it has reached the third or even fourth quarter, a new joiner or a leaver will push the clock back, and the development process will need to start 'ticking' again. Whenever the team's composition changes, the start of a 'new' team is signalled. Existing staff will have anxieties about a new member's competence; a new member will need to learn how to belong – the ground rules.

As manager you need to facilitate this 'forming' process by providing opportunities for personal and professional getting-to-know sessions, for example a meal before a staff meeting. You need to be available and accessible, not judgemental, and observing of the ways in which staff are interacting. This will build trust and security amongst team members. The next step for them is to start to take risks and to challenge each other.

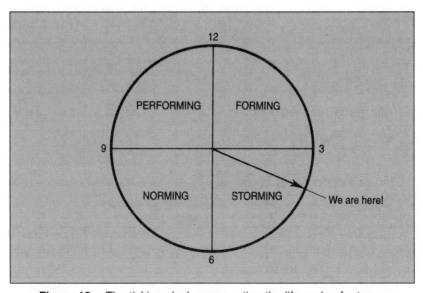

Figure 12.   The ticking clock representing the life cycle of a team.

Confronting conflict

After an initial 'honeymoon' period, it is natural for team members to start asserting themselves, to start negotiating rotas and responsibilities according to their skills and interests. People become concerned with procedures, policies and who sets the agenda, and question decision-making procedures. 'I only take instructions from the manager' and 'They can't tell us to do that' start to typify discussion.

Respect for each individual's contribution, and support in equal measure demonstrated through informal supervision and formal appraisal, are critical to this stage of team building, and time must be put aside by the manager to ensure that they are provided.

Conflict is inevitable in a group, and it leads to healthy discussion and positive solutions, when effectively managed. This is 'storming'. If conflict is avoided, then discussions are put off, leaving everyone feeling frustrated and low. Above all, staff will probably be reluctant to attend and contribute to further meetings.

The manager's skill here is to be an active listener, and to be an assertive chairperson – to ensure that everyone has their say, but that the discussion is moved on. Time should be taken at the outset of the meeting to provide up-to-date information and to clarify expectations of the meeting, in order that discussion remains focused. If staff are able to vent irrelevant frustrations, they only hold up the meeting, and leave feeling bad about using the meeting for that purpose. Such an issue needs to be identified and time set aside elsewhere to deal with it.

Consensus and cooperation

Having worked through some conflict, members of the team are probably now ready and need to experiment with new practices, engage in open debate, and challenge long-standing procedures. This is because members now trust each other, and value the results of working as a combined unit.

Reaching this stage heralds the advent of change. 'We' is heard more often that 'I' or 'You'. Conflicts may still occur but the members now wish to protect group cohesion, and it will be overcome positively.

The manager's role here is to promote cohesion by involving

staff in goal-setting and the development of policy, enabling staff to implement new practices themselves. Then team spirit has been engendered and the process of 'norming' has begun.

Effective team performance

Now all members are making an equal, and equally valued, contribution to the task. Change is anticipated and planned for, and the team embraces it as a new challenge. The team becomes proud of its achievements, and members reacquire their independence as well as their interdependence (see Case Study 5).

The manager is able to relax, and turn his or her attention to the development of other future leaders, to 'Where do we want to go next' in terms of service development. But this phase of team development will last only until a member leaves or a new member joins, and the clock starts to tick again. The manager must be sensitive to the needs of others at this point: 'This wouldn't have happened if Lorraine was still here', and 'Wasn't it great before all the changes', need to be accepted as part of the process, and got through in order that the team moves forward again.

When there is a wholesale change in the team, most members will remember how good the team-building process felt and will be highly motivated to reach effective team performance again.

The Team Manager

On a daily basis, a manager moves from being an administrator to being in direct care of children, and back again. Both manager and team members must adapt to the constant changes in a manager's position in the team.

When in the office, the manager's role can be understood; when she is working directly with children, is she the person in authority? How should team members interact with the manager when she is working with children?

If the team has reached a stage of effective performance, the presence of the manager as one of the team should not present a problem: there is a shared respect and task goals are clear. However, when others in the team are still trying to establish their authority, demonstrate their contribution, fulfil their role, then the manager's presence can cause confusion.

Case Study 5

Nursery teams were asked to look at how they would move around the clock more effectively, and to set themselves a 'challenge'; here are two different approaches:

Nursery A's team challenge is 'communication'. This will entail the following:

- *Listen to one another and allow each staff member to have their say.*
- *Appreciate one another's opinions and value any relevant information that is being passed on.*
- *Learn to compromise in the event of disagreement.*
- *Be more open about criticism. If there is a problem, address the staff member in question and avoid discussing the matter when the person is not there.*

Nursery B's team challenge is:

- *To improve communication within the nursery, particularly between the two areas – upstairs and downstairs. We believe that this will provide increased opportunities for new experiences and self-development for both staff and children.*
- *To work towards increased organisation in the maintenance of the nursery without compromising the care or stimulation of the children. To streamline the 'chores' and encourage people to take joint responsibility for these duties by way of rotas and job lists. The aim is to be constantly reviewing and improving the nursery and increased respect for our environment.*
- *To increase confidence and to support one another in activity planning. To build up resources and establish an index and storage system that enables staff to access resources when needed. To maximise opportunities for new ideas and a wide variety of activities so that staff and children are involved in a fresh and interesting programme each day.*
- *To increase our liaison with other nurseries within the company by way of visits and officer meetings.*
- *To learn more about the community in which we are sited and to build on the relationships with that community.*

However, the manager's participation in day-to-day interactions should not be avoided. It is important to remember that the nursery exists firstly for children, and secondly for parents – both of whom need to see and know the manager.

Some ways in which the manager can add to the performance of the team and stay true to the roles and responsibilities already established are:

- to act as a role model through interacting with children, parents and staff in a professional and authoritative manner;
- to introduce a new activity or new resources, i.e. extend the programme for children;
- to use the time as a training session for a new member of the team.

Equally, to avoid the following would be wise:

- undertaking spot checks on procedures whilst participating;
- automatically taking over a child who is having problems settling;
- intervening in a key-worker–parent dialogue before being asked.

The features of a good team are that it: shares a consistent approach to problems, allows time for its members to participate, and has a system for evaluating progress in dealing with tasks. The manager of a team pulls all this together, and coordinates the work.

Since the aim is to provide a consistent service that is capable of withstanding staff absences, embracing different levels of experience, and coping with the similar problems of different parents and children, the manager needs to be able to rely on staff to deal with matters in a way that is based on common policies and procedures. No one individual can be at a nursery for the full extent of its opening hours, which inevitably leads to a number of staff members dealing with any particular issue. As we have already seen, committing standard procedures to writing can facilitate consistency. Feedback, discussion and review, with the manager acting as coordinator, can take it still further.

This means making time for such dialogue. The manager will need to assess whether immediate support for a staff member or situation is required; or whether the necessary follow-up can take place at the next staff meeting.

In order to move forward together, it is important that as a whole the staff team have the opportunity to share experiences: to consider whether they can all adopt the same approach when faced with a similar situation, and whether a new or revised procedure should be incorporated into the nursery manual.

I referred earlier to the role of a nursery manager being that of a coordinator. In our nurseries, our managers are called Coordinators because of the emphasis we place on teamwork, and its close relationship to quality of service. In the role of a team leader a manager is required to:

- respond to others' needs;
- promote team 'spirit';
- motivate staff;
- allow ideas to be explored;
- enable teams to plan;
- direct/assist in decision-making;
- identify the strengths of each team member and ensure they are utilised;
- offer support;
- provide positive feedback.

Dealing With Conflicts

A manager is expected to recognise when a conflict between two parties is brewing, and to intervene appropriately. Rarely is the wise course of action to let it develop naturally! The signs frequently manifest themselves in the form of destructive criticism, or by somebody refusing to take responsibility, expecting others to solve a problem, or parties breaking into sub-groups rather than wanting to discuss things as a whole or openly sharing the problem.

A manager must also be able to balance confidentiality with the need for knowledge. Conflicts are likely to be sensitive, and in some instances highly personal. Clearly you can respond appropriately only if you have sufficient knowledge of the position of both parties, but you may have to construct your advice on scanty information.

If a potential conflict could affect a child, then the manager should intervene and seek a resolution immediately. No other course of action is consistent with the nursery's primary responsibility being to children, under the provisions of the Children Act.

Strategies that a manager might employ in dealing with conflicts include:

- assertiveness coming from confidence in the culture of mutual respect;
- support and direction in the form of supervision for staff;
- recognition and feedback for the team member involved.

Selling the Nursery

Maintaining occupancy of the nursery in accordance with budgets is fundamental to the ability to deliver the service in the manner intended. Chapter 6 looks at the financial reality of a nursery. However, it is important to appreciate at this point that, because fixed costs are so high, and because staff costs are such a high proportion of total costs, little can be cut out without radically affecting quality of service. If the nursery does not fill, costs are not covered. It is as simple as that.

As a manager you will know that the location of the nursery has been researched, and that there is a local market of parents who are likely to want to view the nursery. It is your job to ensure that each visiting parent gets an accurate picture of the service provided, and that they understand the terms on which a place can be reserved for their child.

In my experience, when there is a complaint about the service, it can be traced back to an initial misunderstanding of the service. In other words the parent's expectation differs from the explanation they heard when visiting at the outset.

The ability on the part of the manager to articulate fundamental principles and philosophies is thus critical. The manager will be expected to have a positive view on, for example, infants in nurseries. Secondly those responsible for showing parents around the nursery must be clear about what service they are selling. It is not helpful, for instance, for a parent to believe they are buying a flexible service if they are required to bring and collect their child at the same time every day.

It will help if the features of the service – those aspects that you feel are important – can be 'translated' into benefits that parents can relate to. For example, the fact that the nursery may employ a comparatively higher ratio of staff to children may not mean anything to a parent. However, if you explain that staff are able to maximise their time with children as there are sufficient assistant staff members to prepare and clear activities, it begins to make sense. The difference between features and benefits is explained fully in Chapter 6.

When parents visit a nursery and appear to have found the service they are looking for – possibly after a long and anxious search – the last thing they wish to discuss is how to extricate themselves from the arrangement. However, the manager *must* be certain that the parents are wholly clear about the terms on which they are booking a place. Any nursery place is expensive, and if a place is being paid for but not used (such as during a notice period), few parents can let it go unnoticed. From the outset the parent must also understand that, although every endeavour will be made to balance the needs of parent and child, it is the nursery's duty to regard the child's needs as paramount.

Issues can arise here, typically over late collections and sick children policies, where parents are under pressure to maximise their working hours. At the same time, they are conscious that nursery policies cannot be compromised.

Working to a Plan

Chapter 6 is devoted to the construction and maintenance of a business plan. This can be a formal document, or drafted on the 'back of an envelope'. However, the benefits of having a framework to guide a manager's work are incalculable. Here we look at the importance in principle of working to a plan.

A manager must know what is expected in the job. There may be specific targets, such as an 85% occupancy at all times, or a 50% staff cost/turnover ratio. Or the targets may be looser, such as 'the manager is responsible for maximising occupancy'. But you need to know what they are. Targets also provide you with a framework for assessing your own performance, and there is no point in denying the inevitable trend towards performance-related pay schemes for managers. This is where an element of salary will be paid 'on commission' for achieving given financial results.

However, targets may not always be financial. They may include, for example, a requirement for the nursery to achieve

Investor in People status within the next 12 months (see Chapter 4); or that the nursery manual is expected to be revised and updated by the end of the year.

As a manager you are entitled to know against what criteria your performance will be assessed in order that you can decide how to prioritise your time and to accomplish tasks in the most efficient way. Such targets also provide you with a framework for reporting, and for assessment of your own accountability.

In more informal situations, working to a plan will mean a continuous dialogue with the nursery owner or management group, to ensure that you communicate over changes in plans and new priorities.

Working to a plan may also imply that training is required in order that you can build the appropriate skills. A classic example here is a manager who has no previous experience of bookkeeping to draw on, and is suddenly responsible for financial reporting in the nursery. A further common example is the daily use of a personal computer.

To achieve the objective of working to a plan, you will need to plan non-contact time carefully, for yourself and also for others who you will need to consult and liaise with, as part of fulfilling your reporting function.

Just as all staff are seriously hampered without a clear entitlement to non child-contact time, which they can devote to planning, observations, liaising with parents, etc., so too must the manager preserve and protect non nursery-contact time. This has resource implications but pays rich dividends in the attitude of others to the managerial role and its importance to the nursery.

Furthering the Quality of Service

In the same way as planning appropriate activities for children relies on careful observation and record-keeping of development to date, so too developing the quality of the service as a whole requires a system to be in place for knowing how the nursery performs in terms of current quality criteria. There are a number of levels on which the nursery as a whole is expected to perform:

- against the nursery registration criteria set out by the local authority;

- against the promises made to parents though the nursery con-tract and promotional literature, and what they have been told;
- against recognised contemporary thinking about children's entitlement, i.e. state-of-the-art childcare.

There are many different schemes for measuring quality of care and education in nursery settings, and there are several schemes under development. The best known is probably that adopted by the National Children's Bureau in *Day Nurseries at a Crossroads* (Vernon and Smith 1994). This scheme was the Pre-Five Environment Quality Rating Scale, developed at Morag House College in 1991. This takes a developmental approach to quality, providing targets rather than absolute measurements. The scale has been criticised, however, for not capturing the overall atmos-phere and warmth of nursery settings – the quality of adult/child interactions and the intimacy of infant care. The scale is being developed to incorporate children aged 0–3 years.

Other schemes have taken a process management approach, rather than looking at outcomes for children. Examples are those from the Department of Health (DoH 1991) and the Thomas Coram Research Unit (1996).

Particular interest groups have developed 'kitemarks' designed to indicate a higher standard of service. Examples are the Pre-School Playgroups Accreditation Scheme (1994) (now called the Pre-School Learning Alliance), and the Childcare Association's Code of Practice (1991).

The proliferation of quality observation schemes suggests that there is a general consensus around a need for 'quality' to be something in excess of the minimum standards required under the Children Act. Against a background of government deregulation it is more likely that parents, too, will seek non-statutory yard-sticks by which they can be assured of quality.

The question will continue to be whether quality is absolute, or a standard that is derived from the objectives of the setting itself. This debate aside, a manager should be in a position of knowing what aspects of service need attention and development.

Observation alone, however, will not improve the service and there needs to be a system in place for taking action on the obser-vations made. My experience with our own nurseries has been that when this process was regarded as an 'audit' by central office staff, it was less effective than it has been more recently, when it became a quality 'observation'. The observation is undertaken by staff themselves and is a rotated responsibility. The monthly observation is discussed with a view to the issues being resolved within the staff team. Only if additional resources are needed, or if policy needs to be reviewed or training is required, should central office now need to be involved. The staff team, led by the manager, owns and is responsible for delivering the quality of service required. The standard of quality is implicit in the observation schedule and system employed.

Because they are carried out by nursery staff, such observations carry the added advantage of being easily discussed with parents, who are then able to take a more holistic view of the nursery than in the delivery of a service to their child alone. An 'audit' undertaken by 'Head Office' might preclude their involvement, or raise anxieties around the need for additional inspection.

Quite apart from various methods of identifying the quality of service as a whole, much work has been taking place over the last few years on curriculum development for under-fives. The Effective Early Learning (EEL) Project (Worcester College of Higher Education 1994) looks at the way in which children learn, and uses a ten-dimensional framework for assessing the quality of educational provision in any setting (the Pascal/Bertram Quality Framework – see Figure 13):

> 'The Pascal/Bertram Quality Evaluation Framework has drawn extensively on the views of practitioners, parents and children in a range of settings and on an informed understanding of research about how young children learn. There is therefore an emphasis on the importance of the social context of learning and, in particular, an emphasis on the importance of the staff in establishing this context. This reflects our belief that learning only takes place when young children have positive relationships with those with whom they are interacting. . . . Within this framework, ten dimensions or aspects of quality may be identified. These dimensions represent the factors highlighted by the many early childhood educators we have worked with over the last three years as significantly affecting the quality of their provision. They are not intended to be an exhaustive list but we believe they provide a broad overview of the quality of educational provision in any setting.'

Quality in Diversity (Early Childhood Education Forum 1996) provides a value-based framework for sourcing everything that goes on in a nursery, for babies through to children aged 8 years.

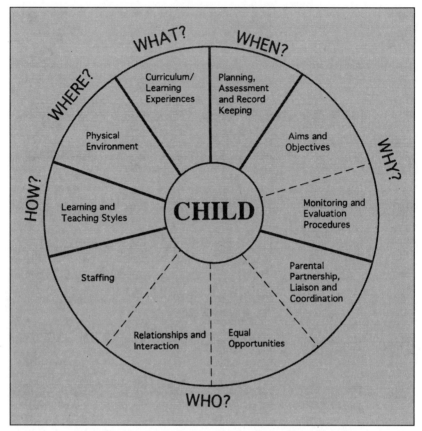

Figure 13. The ten dimensions of the EEL project.

As part of the government's nursery voucher scheme, the Schools Curriculum Assessment Authority (SCAA) has published *Desirable Learning Outcomes for Children* as they reach compulsory school age; i.e. a guide to curriculum planning for pre-school settings.

Such initiatives receive a lot of publicity and parents are generally aware of them. A nursery manager needs to be in a position to respond to questions, and to justify the nursery's curriculum alongside new educational thinking.

Planning Staff Shifts

A well-run nursery relies on everyone knowing the routine and the part they play in achieving it. Conversely, each and every member of staff must understand the implications and consequences for others of not cooperating and working with the routines as set out.

Given that most nurseries open for more hours each day than staff are required to work, there is likely to be a shift pattern, requiring a change of shifts for each individual on a weekly or monthly basis. Each member of staff needs to know the routine of each shift – the ebb and flow of each shift – and the differing tasks that need to be accomplished. Most importantly they need to know how one shift flows into another. This raises a number of important issues:

- the sense of responsibility that all staff must share in the whole nursery and for all children, whilst acknowledging particular strengths within the staff team;
- the need to engage children as often as possible throughout the day by having a rolling programming of activities on offer;
- the importance of targeting some activities for particular age or ability groups, as well as for mixed age or ability groups;
- compatibility of activities taking place alongside one another;
- planning in advance to alert staff to their responsibilities to consider how parents can be involved to prepare necessary resources, and to involve children in the planning process.

In any rota of activities there will be room for improvement, and although some 'deviations' can be planned for – holiday and sick absences, new children settling – you can never adequately allow for unexpected human 'failure'. Examples of the latter are expectations of new staff that are too high, personal ups and downs, lack of familiarisation time, children's moods, parents' demands.

Rota planning probably leans towards being an art rather than a science, and the target needs to be around making it work for most of the people, most of the time. We have learned that:

- Rotas must be given time and a chance to work, so stick with them for a sensible period.
- Provided that an appropriate range of activities is available to children, not every area of the nursery, nor every opportunity in the nursery, need always be available.

- All areas of the nursery in which planned activities are taking place must be supervised by staff allocated to that area.
- Care routines must never be compromised.
- Children can be engaged in planning, preparing for and tidying up activities.

The results of this practical approach to rota planning include the following:

- Quality of staff interaction with children is maintained.
- Staff gain fulfilment from the (fewer) activities they can properly engage in.
- Staff are less concerned with 'policing' and are able to release more time for children and parents.
- Children gain a positive attitude with regard to clutter and waste, and efficient space utilisation.

Planning human resources is dealt with in depth in Chapter 2.

Examples of responsibilities where a 3-shift day is worked

Early 1

06.45   Read and add to message book
        Prepare room and activities
07.00   Welcome children
        Engage children in table-top activity
08.10   Tidy-up time
08.15   Sit children down for breakfast
        Engage in play children who are not eating breakfast
09.00   After nappy change etc., engage children in play
09.30   Outside play
10.30   Tidy up nursery/reset tables
11.10   Break
12.10   Lunch – sit down to receive key children
12.40   Prepare sleeping area(s)/washing
13.00   Settle sleepers
13.30   Nursery paperwork (activity plans)
14.45   Home – pass on relevant information

Early 2

06.45	Read and add to message book
	Prepare room and activities
07.00	Prepare bottles and breakfast trolley
	Engage children in malleable and painting area
08.10	Tidy up
08.15	Collect breakfast and sit with children to offer breakfast
09.00	Set up an activity
10.30	Spend time with rabbit
11.10	Lunch break
12.10	Lunch time – receive children and sit with key children
12.45	Take children to bathroom and then to sleeping area(s)
13.00	Settle sleepers/sort washing
14.30	Pass any relevant information to middle/late shift staff
14.45	Home

Middle (Baby Room)

09.00	Read and add to message book
	Take children to bathroom and change nappies
	Tidy bathroom
09.30	Activities
12.00	Tidy
12.10	Sit down for lunch with children
12.30	Break
13.30	Engage younger children in play
14.30	Pass on or collect any information/other staff
14.45	Offer story
15.15	Plan outing/activity etc.
16.15	Tea time
16.45	Take children to the bathroom – wash hands etc.
	Tidy bathroom
17.00	Go home

Late 1

11.00	Read and add to message book – take over from Early 1
11.40	Take over outside
12.05	Take children to bathroom
12.10	Lunch time – sit with key children
12.45	Set up activities
	Wait for children to come out of bathroom and then involve them in activities
13.30	Go for lunch
14.30	Come back from lunch
	Collect information from Early Shift
	Re-spruce activities, overseeing children engaged in inside play
15.15	Be involved with outings or general play
16.05	Take children to bathroom
16.15	Tea time
16.45	Tea time finished
	Prepare children for going home
	Welcome parents
17.30	Tidy up creative play materials (paint, water, sand etc.)
18.00	Tidy up nursery with children who are left, and also continue to interact and play
19.00	Go home

Late 2

11.00	Read and add to message book – gain feedback from staff
11.10	Take over and continue from Early 2 – encourage play
11.40	Tidy up, with children's help
11.50	Offer story and/or singing
12.05	Send children to bathroom – toilet and washing hands
	Help middle shift to prepare children for lunch
12.10	Lunch time – sit with key children
12.40	Take children to bathroom and stay to tidy bathroom when they have gone, then go back to main room
13.30	Go for lunch break
14.30	Information exchange with early shift
14.45	Offer outside play
15.15	Plan outings, special activities etc.

16.15   Tea time – sit with children
16.45   Clear tables and tidy kitchen
17.00   Back to room and play
17.30   Spend time with nursery pets
18.00   With the children who are left, tidy up outside area, shelves, book corner etc.
19.00   Update message book and go home

Late 3

10.00   Read and add to message book
10.05   Offer story and/or songs
10.30   Offer outside play
11.40   Tidy up with children
11.50   Continue tidying up, and prepare tables for lunch with cook and children
12.05   Bathroom
12.10   Lunch time – sit with children
12.30   Lunch break
13.30   Offer activity
14.30   Relieve early shift upstairs
          As children wake, check nappies and send downstairs
16.15   Tea (surface tidy and spruce)
16.45   Encourage children to play inside
17.30   Offer story and songs
18.00   Add to message book and go home

Communication

The principal ways we communicate are by the spoken word and in writing.

The spoken word

Good verbal communication is a two-way process. The speaker gives the listeners the opportunity to ask questions and make comments about what has been said in order to clarify.

The objective of verbal communication is to give a message in such a way as to be easily understood by the listeners – and to be sure that they understand it. There are, however, a number of barriers that get in the way, distorting or even shutting out the messages we try to send.

Barriers include physical distractions such as noise, temperature and lighting, and emotional distractions such as personal prejudices, experience, assumptions, or values and beliefs. Certain words can cause us to stop listening altogether. This can happen when people are moralising, threatening, criticising or just using jargon. So a good starting point in improving communication is to think about these barriers and prepare your communications with them in mind. Talk to people in an atmosphere free of interruptions and use words that don't rub people up the wrong way. Whilst you can't do much about other people's emotions, you can do something about your own. Stay calm and neutral. If you sense emotional barriers in others, either keep your conversation brief and to the point, or postpone it.

Speaking effectively

It is generally believed that each of the following elements has a specific value in transmitting the 'true' message:

- words 7%
- tone 35%
- non-verbal or body language 58%.

You may disagree with these percentages, but think about it for a moment. You have complete control over the words that you use. You have less control over the tone as your emotion begins to take over. Trying saying the phrase 'Where did you go last night?' without emphasising any of the words. Repeat it, putting an emphasis on the first word, then again, this time emphasising the word 'you'. Three different 'true' messages will be conveyed to the listener and they will respond accordingly.

You have virtually no control over the non-verbal body language. Subconsciously your body will reveal what you really mean and think. If you sit with your arms and legs crossed, this is a defensive posture and indicates a hostile attitude towards the other person and/or the message. Sitting with your arms folded with your thumbs up shows a superior attitude. Leaning forward indicates interest or intimidation. People who rest their chin on one hand, and have a finger in or near their mouth, need reassurance. Those who rub their chin are thinking or making a decision and will not be listening to you, so stop talking. These are gestures, intentional movements, and should not be confused with body language. You may be able to control your body language at the beginning of a conversation, but the more you become involved, the more your subconscious will take over.

To back up the importance of body language at the beginning of a conversation, it should be noted that, of information relayed, 87% is via the eyes, 9% is via the ears, and 4% is via the other senses (taste, touch, etc.).

A vital part of speaking effectively is being sure people understand what you mean. This is best done by asking a question. Never say 'Do you understand?' as this puts the onus on the listener and, rather than appear stupid, they will probably say 'yes'. If you say 'Have I explained that satisfactorily?' then the responsibility rests with you – the listener does not feel threatened and can answer honestly.

The following are the categories of questions that can be used depending upon the type of information you want in return:

- *Elaboration questions* – for information of a general nature:
  'Tell me about . . .'
  'Is there anything more?'
  'Would you elaborate on that please.'

- *Specification questions* – asking for more detailed information:
  'What precisely did she say?'
  'When was the last time this happened?'

- *Feeling questions* – when you want to know the emotional effect of something:
  'What did you feel when it happened?'
  'How do you feel when people are aggressive towards you?'

- *Opinion questions* – most people hold opinions about things and welcome the opportunity to express them:
  'What do you like about your present job?'
  'What do you least like about your job?'
  'What would you like that you don't have?'

- *Behavioural questions* – past behaviour is a good indicator of further behaviour:

'How would you usually deal with a situation like this?'
'What did you do the last time this happened?'
'How did you react when . . . ?'

Listening

Listening is a key part of speaking effectively. It is not enough just to concentrate and to understand; you need to let the other person know you have been listening.

The simplest way of indicating that you have listened to the speaker is by employing reflective techniques. Reflection is a form of summary of what has been said. It demonstrates empathy with the speaker.

Our responses fall into one of three types:

- apathy or dismissiveness – showing lack of interest in what has been said;
- sympathy – sharing the feeling of others, allowing their problem to become your problem;
- showing that you appreciate the other person's feelings or point of view without becoming involved or agreeing with them.

Imagine that someone says to you 'I am a bit down at the moment, my grandfather died yesterday. He was a lovely old chap and a real companion. I am going to miss him.'

- Apathetic response: 'Really, anyway, as I was saying . . .'
- Sympathetic response: 'I know how you must feel, I felt dreadful for weeks after my aunt passed away last year.'
- Empathetic response: 'You must feel very upset.'

The written word

Many people feel uncomfortable with the written word. They put off writing reports and proposals and they dash off poorly conceived letters because they have not been taught to write in a way that is useful at work. The value of logically constructed, accurate, comprehensible and interesting written communication is considerable. If you realise that this is not one of your strengths, this section will hopefully help you feel more confident about putting pen to paper (or fingers to the keyboard).

The general rules about writing are the same regardless of the type of document you are producing, so it may be helpful to look at those rules first and follow up with a discussion of the different forms the writing may take. Written communications should be clear, readable, relevant and informative. To achieve this, the following guidelines should be observed.

Personal Well-being

'Stress management' is a common phrase today, but I prefer to think of it in terms of 'personal effectiveness' or 'handling pressure'. The word 'stress' has mainly negative connotations but actually there are many positive aspects to it. Sports people and actors rely on the increased flow of adrenalin to bring out their best performances. Nursery managers chairing important staff or parent meetings also experience feelings of excitement, nervousness and heightened awareness before and during their performance. They also feel drained and exhausted afterwards. This is all quite normal and should not cause concern. In itself, stress is not harmful, but it is best to avoid unnecessary pressures, to know how to cope with them if they do arise and to recognise the symptoms of too much stress.

Pressures of time

Many people worry about the fact that there are not enough hours in a day, and it may seem worse if you are, effectively, a one-person business having to do everything yourself.

It is possible to introduce some routine into your work without losing the flexibility that the nursery needs. If done thoughtfully, this will enable you to optimise the time spent doing what you really want to do, rather than worrying about administrative or operational details. You will also still have energy left for the other things you value in your life.

In any occupation there are tasks that must be done, those that should be done if possible, and those that would be satisfying or fun to do but which are not essential to the progress and success of the nursery. If you make a list of jobs to do at the beginning of each week or at the start of a day, this is one of several ways of categorising what, when and how you should tackle your work.

From the tasks that *must* be done, identify those that have to be done quickly and those that need some time and thought spent on them. Check that 'urgent' tasks really do have to be done – I am always intrigued by how many so-called urgent matters do not really need to be attended to until tomorrow and how many actually become obsolete. If anyone tells me that a task is urgent, I try to establish with them an actual time for completion so that I know what the deadline is.

When you have decided which jobs are important and which are urgent, you then allocate the necessary time to them. A good diary or daily planning sheet is useful in helping you give priorities to the demands on your time. It is also worth thinking about the time of day when you work best (i.e. morning or afternoon). When do you think most clearly, find it easiest to make decisions, and produce good written work?

When you have decided which is your best time, try to arrange your work programme around that and leave the routine, less important, matters to your least effective part of the day. Some of my colleagues who find it very difficult to wake up in the morning appreciate not having to rush into work early. Your timetable is more flexible when you have control over your day.

One way of reducing the feeling that you have to be working at full speed all day long is to pace yourself and vary the types of task you work on. Do not rush at everything indiscriminately – pause, put matters into perspective and introduce a change of pace into your work pattern. For example, intersperse the 'easy' piece of work with a few routine tasks such as the filing, making some phone calls, or treating yourself to a cup of coffee when you have finished a particularly difficult task. It is difficult to handle freedom and flexibility, if you have been used to a strict regime as a team member up until now.

Staying healthy

There are many pressures on nursery managers to succumb to an unhealthy life style. Invitations to seminars and meetings, tight deadlines, worrying about cash flow and future bookings, and feelings of isolation and helplessness all contribute to stress. You have to recognise where and when stress occurs. Try to identify and write down occasions, people and times that regularly increase your tension. Is it money, deadlines, lack of time, particular people? Just the act of knowing where the problems are helps you to find a solution, an alternative way of doing things.

When you really are under an unreasonable amount of stress, the physical symptoms should alert you to the situation. You may feel tense, have constant headaches or sore throats, suffer from digestive problems, keep going hot and cold, notice that your hands are trembling, and generally feel not well. You may also feel different. You may be aware that you feel panicky, always on the defensive and generally depressed. Your behaviour will change – perhaps you are becoming aggressive, relying on drink, cigarettes or drugs to calm you down, and you may become accident prone.

All of these signs mean that you have to stand back and take stock of the situation, and take the necessary steps towards a healthier way of living. Except in extreme medical cases, you may be able to heal yourself with some simple resolutions.

Eat sensibly, exercise properly and rest well

It is tempting to keep on working if you are busy and not have breaks for lunch or a mid-morning cup of coffee. Part of pacing yourself properly is to know when to take breaks to rest your brain, to move your limbs and have a change of surroundings. Taking lunch does not place you under an obligation to stop for a full hour or to eat an enormous meal washed down with alcohol. I very much dislike the 'working lunch' (or breakfast or dinner come to that); I am sure that asking the brain and digestive system to work at full speed at the same time leads to indigestion of both head and stomach, and under-performance in both.

Some kind of exercise is beneficial to everyone. This does not mean rushing to the squash court once every six months to prove that you are still young and active. Exercise should be regular, within your capabilities, and you should always warm up and 'warm down' before and after any physical activity. Much serious illness in busy people is due to irregular strenuous exercise without preparing the body adequately for the unaccustomed exertion.

The body needs rest as well as exercise if the correct balance is to be maintained. Some people need more sleep than others but, however long you need, make sure that you have enough. There will always be times when circumstances mean you have to work extremely hard for a few days, and this may result in only a few hours' sleep each night during that period. The body can easily cope with this if you are fit, but will react badly if it becomes a regular occurrence.

Have regular check-ups

This is particularly important as you get older or if you have a history of illness. If you object in principle to belonging to one of the private health schemes, your doctor will be pleased to give you a general examination to test that everything is well.

In addition to modern medicine, you may wish to consult practitioners of complementary or alternative medicine. For example, if you suffer from back pain, you are as likely to find relief from a chiropractor as from a doctor. The nature of nursery work places heavy stresses on the body – for instance, lifting heavy toddlers on to a changing mat many times in a day, or bending to pick up babies. You might consider learning the Alexander Technique, which teaches you to 'fine tune' your body, how to bring it back into balance. To what extent you use these complementary methods will depend on your own beliefs.

There is also much you can introduce into the nursery to relieve such physical stress on staff, such as adult-height chairs for sitting in to receive babies from parents, and steps to enable toddlers to reach the changing surface themselves.

Learn to relax

Take regular bouts of proper relaxation and build them into your day. This is a time for deep unwinding, not just five minutes sitting at your desk with a cup of tea. You can learn how to meditate or devote time to a personal way of relaxing such as walking, music or sport. The time set aside for this must be preserved – and must not be the first thing to be sacrificed as soon as work builds up.

The office

For people who have not been used to running an office or doing all the administrative work themselves, the new routines and details may prove a source of stress. For an office to provide a sound support for you and your work, it is worth spending time setting up the systems that will actually help you and not just create frustration.

If you really hate office work but cannot afford any help yet, arrange a routine so that you do the filing, type up the invoices, update the accounts and check the stationery supplies regularly and efficiently. In that way you will spend as little time as is necessary on these tasks. They have to be done, and you can get yourself into all sorts of trouble, operational and legal, if they are neglected. If you are in a situation that makes it extremely difficult to get office work done – for example in a small nursery the manager may be included in the ratio of staff to children – you could investigate the possibility of having a business administration student from the local college come in to help one day a week. This provides them with a useful placement, and you with an identified time for routine office work to be dealt with.

I would emphasise the importance of the design of your workplace, particularly in relation to the way it affects you physically. An office should be well ventilated but not too cold. Also, if you have computers and photocopiers in a smallish space, do not allow them to overheat.

Many people who operate computer keyboards have not learned to type on a traditional typewriter. While this does not affect their ability to operate the machine, it may mean that they do not know how to sit properly, or understand where their hands and arms should be in relation to the keyboard. There are increasing numbers of cases of repetitive strain injury (RSI) being reported among people who use keyboards often. This is a very painful inflammation of the joints, usually the wrists, elbows and up to the shoulders and neck in serious cases. It occurs through repeating particular actions over a long period of time, and when it first appears many patients and doctors think it is rheumatism. For anyone who uses a keyboard, the advice is to make sure you take regular breaks, not only from straining your eyes looking at the screen, but also from repeating the action of striking the keys. Stop every twenty minutes or so and do something else for a short while. In extreme cases, sufferers may not regain the full use of their hands if they do not heed the first warning pains.

Another common factor in RSI cases is that keyboards are often too high in front of the operator. Ideally your shoulders should be down and your hands and elbows in a straight line, parallel to the floor and level with the keyboard. This means buying a good chair.

Be fit for life – maintaining the balance

One way to minimise the negative aspects of stress is to strike the right personal balance between work, home and leisure. This balance will be different for every individual and may change during the various phases of your life, so it is worth reviewing your priorities from time to time.

During your first two or three years as a manager you will probably be tempted to become totally immersed in your work. It is at this time that even the most understanding partners and friends will find that their patience is sorely tested. Most people will recognise your need to build up the nursery, but your true friends will also persuade you to honour your holiday commitments, join the local gym or take up photography – or anything that will keep your work in perspective. Most importantly, discuss what is happening with the people with whom you are most deeply involved. They will also be picking up the phone when your staff ring on a Sunday night to say they are sick.

Managing Yourself and Others

Analysing your objectives will lead to a priority order of tasks. The next step is to look at *your own* strengths and weaknesses in relation to these tasks. Remember, you are doing two things: starting up or maintaining a childcare project, and secondly, securing its permanence and stability by treating it as a *business*.

There are three areas in which leadership and management need to be apparent:

- technical authority;
- managing people;
- managing the business.

How would you rate your abilities against the following list, taken from the National Westminster Bank's *Guide to the Preparation of a Business Plan*?

I am self-disciplined and do not let things drift.
I have the full support of my family.
I am ready to put in 7 days a week, if necessary.
I can get on well with people.

I can make careful decisions.
I can cope under stress.
I do not give up when the going gets tough.
I can learn from mistakes.
I can take advice.
I am patient, and I expect a long haul.
I can motivate people.
I am in good health.
I am enthusiastic.
I know about the risks.
I have specific aims.

In order to plan what additional *human* resources you need, you must first decide what you are going to do as a manager, and the role you will play in relation to others. You will be making a broad transition of attitudes from acting on instructions to directing and supervising the carrying out of instructions you have given. You will be in a position of authority, requiring assertiveness and evaluation skills, rather than compliance and response. Although you will retain accountability for the actions of others, you will not be *doing* everything. You will start to rely on others to come up with ideas, and then assess them and make decisions. And you will become a listener and supporter of others. This last quality is often the most difficult for a new manager to learn. Nursery managers are exceptional in this role, it being a central part of the training and experience as a nursery nurse.

Managing yourself

It is hard to see how anyone can seriously expect to become an effective business manager until they can first manage their own activities.

There are three aspects to managing yourself that need to be kept under regular review and have a major impact on the ability of the rest of your staff to be able to perform. The first is managing your own time – vital if you are to win back the opportunity to think and plan; the second is managing meetings, or other people's time – vital if your team is going to have to change to do their job effectively; the third is effective communication.

Managing time

Most owner–managers have a false impression of how they use their time and how it affects their performance. There is a strong body of research that suggests that a typical MD could improve his or her output by at least 105% and save time by as much as 20–30 hours in a typical working week. A prize such as having an 8- or 9-day week at your disposal is surely worth a modest investment of time and energy. There are many time management systems on the market, but you can realise many of the benefits yourself immediately without any expense.

Step 1

Have a daily and weekly 'to do' list. Most senior people in business have a diary scheduling meetings and the like but do not have lists of key tasks to be completed each day and each week. It follows that, without a set of daily objectives, key priorities cannot be established, nor can you commit to driving hard to achieve those objectives.

Step 2

Establish the key priorities. A manager's day is made up of different types of priorities:

- 'A' priorities are highly essential activities that must be completed or progressed substantially.
- 'B' priorities are less essential activities that can be deferred because the time element is less critical and the impact on job performance is lower.
- 'C' priorities are non-essential activities that can be scrapped, screened out, handled by other people or handled at low-priority times.
- 'X' priorities are activities that require immediate attention. There may be queries, requests for information, crises and emergencies, boss demands or interruptions. You can have 'AX', 'BX' or 'CX' priorities.

One of the golden rules of time management is based on the Pareto or 80/20 rule. This suggests that 80% of your performance will come from 20% of your activities, and 20% of your performance will come from 80% of your activities.

When you assess your own time usage and your own performance in the day, you will find that the majority of your time has been spent on lower priority work. Log the following:

- For each activity calculate the time you spent on it.
- For each activity assign an ABCX priority.
- Work out the total time spent on ABCX priorities as a percentage of the total day.
- Ask a very frank question about your 'A' priority activities. 'Did I achieve what I intended to achieve?'
- Estimate the time you could have saved, by better discipline and control, on each low-priority activity.
- Make a judgement about your achievement on the day: how much 'continuous' time you spent on your top-priority work and how much 'total' time you could have devoted to high-priority work if you had exercised better control and discipline.

When you go through this assessment you may find that you are not spending enough time on your top-priority work in order to achieve, and that the majority of time (which could be as high as 60% or 70%) will be spent on low-priority work of which you could have saved at least 20% by better control and discipline.

Review how you spend your time

This is a simple technique whereby you sum the total amount of time (in percentages) you spend in certain categories of activities. Typical C categories are: meetings, telephone, correspondence, project work, report writing, reading, etc. Each manager will have different categories and different times, but managers usually find they spend at least 40–50% of a typical day in some sort of meeting.

If you made an assessment of the amount of time you could save by 'crisper' management of these activities, you would find that your time saving could be between 20% and 30%. The three priority areas for time saving and better self-management are delegation, meetings, and personal organisation.

Keeping a log

You can make a start on improving your time management by keeping a daily log for three or four days, reviewing how you spent your time – and look for ways to save time, improve performance or delegate tasks.

Managing meetings

Meetings consume between one and three days of a business week. It follows that anything that can be done to make them more effective must be good news. Meetings are vital. They are a forum for exchanging ideas and gaining fresh thinking, a way to communicate complex information, a way to gain consensus and commitment to key decisions. Unfortunately most people see most meetings as a complete waste of time – including the person who called the meeting! The following are some points to help make your meetings more effective.

Define the purpose

Know exactly what you expect to achieve. Meetings without set objectives demotivate people. The purpose might be to inform staff of new initiatives/procedures (in many instances a memo would be a quicker, cheaper and just as efficient a way of doing this); it might be to identify and resolve a particular problem, to review progress and give people an opportunity to express their views. Asking yourself what would happen if the meeting was not held is a great help in defining its objectives.

Decide who should attend

The fewer participants the better if the meeting is going to achieve its objectives in a reasonable length of time. However, research has shown that larger groups often come up with sounder decisions than individuals or a small number of people – but take much longer to do so.

Ensure everyone prepares properly

A meeting is much less stressful if all the participants have prepared in advance, yourself included. If possible, circulate beforehand a note giving notice of the meeting with the agenda items. The note should state the purposes of the meeting and probable duration (to give people a chance to organise the rest of their day). An agenda is vital for any meeting. It acts as the control device, establishing order and sequence, assigning tasks and providing guidelines for the timing of each item. If a meeting is called on the spur of the moment, it should still have an agenda, even if it is just jotted down on the back of an envelope. An agenda sent in advance gives people a chance to do their homework.

If participants need to have absorbed specific information before they can discuss an item, it is much better to send this out well in advance since nothing wastes more time than people sitting reading during a meeting.

Be a good listener

People who chair meetings need to listen more carefully than anyone else in the group since it is their job to make sure the real point of someone's contribution isn't being missed. They need to pick the right moment to move on, clarify points when people are getting in a muddle, and summarise all the views when it is time to push for a decision.

Involve all the participants

People are likely to feel far more committed to the meeting and decisions reached if they have had a chance to say their piece. And, indeed, people should not be at the meeting unless they have something to contribute. It is the leader's task to ensure that everyone has a chance to participate.

Use open-ended questions to get people to talk (questions that start with words such as how, what, why, when – these are impossible to answer with a Yes or No).

Make positive noises throughout the session ('Anybody add to that?' 'Any more?') to encourage the shy. Check round the group ('Let's see where we all stand on that; Terri, you first') – this not only forces people to speak but also generally motivates the meeting.

Closed questions (those that begin with do, can, are, which – these are usually answerable with a Yes or a No) can be used to bring the talkative to a halt.

Keep the meeting on course

Red herrings and ramblings are the chief dangers when you are trying to stay on course and keep to time limits. There are polite ways to stem the speaker's flow: cough, lean forward, raise your eyebrows, or use the more positive 'We're getting off the point aren't we?' Don't be too tolerant with people who regularly take the meeting off at a tangent or you'll lose the respect of the others who want to see your hand firmly on the wheel.

Control aggression

Conflict can be healthy in that it encourages new ideas and new ways of solving problems. It is the chairperson's job to ensure that everyone has a fair say and a fair hearing even if they are disagreeing. However, some control may need to be exercised if things are getting particularly ugly or someone with strong views is being very vocal.

You must avoid taking sides or apportioning blame – this always provokes an argument, and the chairperson who loses his or her temper loses credibility in the process.

Check that everyone understands

You need to know both that the rest of the group is not at cross-purposes with the speaker, and that they understand what he or she is trying to convey. So check assumptions by asking following questions: 'So you mean that if we improve X we'll get better results from Y?' Make a habit of providing a verbal summary of what has been said.

Decide on action

The purpose of meetings is not to impose decisions but to reach decisions by consensus. Once decisions have been made, remind everyone of what they are, define clearly how they are to be acted upon, by whom and by when.

Memories being short, it is essential to produce minutes (or at least some notes) of every meeting, if for no other reason than to prevent subsequent arguments over who was responsible for what. Another of the chairperson's tasks is to ensure that this is done, although he or she may well prefer to delegate minute-taking to someone else in the group.

The minutes should be brief and strictly factual, describing what happened without distortion or comment, sticking to suggestions and proposals with the names of the people who made them, actions agreed and the name of the person responsible for each action.

Minutes of a meeting should be sent out within a couple of days, especially if there are a number of actions to be carried out. If it is not possible to do this, then a summary may be made of the actions agreed and copies distributed immediately after the meeting. A sheet similar to the one shown in Figure 14 may be used as a simple way of recording actions during a meeting.

Make sure decisions are implemented

If the meeting was worth having, the decisions are worth implementing, so your job doesn't stop when the meeting finishes. You need to monitor progress, which may involve holding a follow-up meeting, asking for interim reports or carrying out day-to-day checks.

Conclusion

There are three interrelated sets of needs that a nursery manager will have to satisfy: task needs, team needs, and individual needs.

MEETING			Date:	
Action Ref:	Action	By whom	By when	Date completed
Chairperson's signature:				

Figure 14. Summary of actions.

Task needs

The difference between a team and a random crowd is that the team has some common purpose or goal. Without this common objective, it would not stick together as a group. If a team does not achieve the required result or output, it will become frustrated.

Organisations have a task to provide a service, to cover costs, or even just to survive. So anyone who manages others has to achieve results.

> **TASK-ORIENTED BEHAVIOUR**
>
> - Agree objective
> - Plan and allocate resources
> - Make decisions
> - Control progress
> - Review and evaluate

Team needs

The group must be held together. People need to work in a co-ordinated fashion in the same direction. Teamwork will ensure that the team contribution is greater than the sums of its parts. Conflict within the team must be used effectively: argument can lead to new ideas, or to tension and lack of cooperation.

> **TEAM-ORIENTED BEHAVIOUR**
>
> - Select the right people
> - Communicate with them
> - Encourage
> - Harmonise
> - Use humour
> - Coordinate

Individual needs

Within working groups, individuals also have their own set of motivational needs: the need to know what their responsibilities are, how they will be judged, how well they are doing. They need an opportunity to show their potential, take on responsibilities and receive recognition for good work.

> ## INDIVIDUAL-ORIENTED BEHAVIOUR
> - Trust and respect
> - Listen
> - Identify training needs
> - Appraise
> - Delegate
> - Develop
> - Motivate
> - Recognise and praise

The manager's job must be to satisfy all three areas of need by achieving the task, building the team and satisfying individual needs. If managers concentrate only on tasks, for example in going all out for achieving output whilst neglecting the training and motivations of their people, they may do very well in the short term. Eventually, however, those people will give less than they know they are capable of. Similarly, neglecting the task will not get the maximum contribution from employees. They will lack the real sense of achievement that comes from accomplishing the task.

Nurseries need to give some attention to their internal communication. Staff tend to be in highly motivated small teams, spending a lot of time together at work and socially. As the nursery grows in numbers, sheer size will start to crack the foundations of this group, and the introduction of new people without the original motivation will change the flavour of relationships. It is at this point that the manager will consciously have to introduce ways and means of getting the team together and keep them facing the right way. Involving your team in the preparation of a business plan can, in itself, be a good way of providing coordination to a growing business.

It is amazing how many business people expect a team to work without any practice. After all, it presumably doesn't work this way for a football team. The way to build up a team is to find many formal and informal ways of bringing them together: cascade briefing, social events, special project teams, happy hours. Fun is actually quite compatible with profit. The importance of informal contact between people, as a way of building productive networks, cannot be overemphasised, but again it won't take place without the mechanism to make it happen.

Appendix to Chapter 3

Language

The written word in business should be simple and straightforward. Many people think that reports and letters have to be written in a different language from the spoken word, but this usually leads to complex sentences and the misuse of words. If you have any problems writing a sentence or paragraph, try saying it aloud. This usually helps to clarify your thoughts.

Although you should always be aware of the person who will be reading what you write, and so use the appropriate words and way of presenting the material, you do not have to use a different kind of English for each type of reader. Your aim is clarity. You are not trying to bewilder or mystify the reader or make life difficult for yourself.

- *Be clear.* Do not allow room for ambiguity or wrong assumptions. For example the following sentence could have two meanings: 'The mother told the member of staff she had made a mistake.' Who made the mistake?
- *Keep it short and simple.* As a writer you are aiming at clarity of expression, balance of ideas and arguments, and interest in what has been written. You should therefore keep sentences and paragraphs short and simple.

  It is advisable to break long sentences down into shorter ones to avoid overusing punctuation. As a sentence grows in length, the rate of reading and comprehension slows down.

  Do not use many words when a few will do, or complicated phrases to express a simple idea. For example, 'in the event that we are in a position to undertake' can be expressed as, 'if we can', and 'endeavour to ascertain' can be expressed as 'try to find out'.

  It is generally easier to read statements that use the active voice rather the passive voice. For example, 'It was declared by John' is better as 'John said', and 'The undersigned was not telephoned by your assistant' can be 'Your assistant did not phone me'.

- *Keep jargon in its place.* You may be able to use technical words for some readers but you may have to explain them to others. Do not resort to jargon unless it is appropriate to the audience. Generally, your technical words and phrases will be incomprehensible to anyone apart from your staff (e.g. 'Christian's gross motor skills are underdeveloped').
- *Avoid clichés.* For example: 'At this moment in time the general standard of English leaves much to be desired, but it goes without saying that at the end of the day it will all come out in the wash!'
- *Use punctuation to help the reader.* Punctuation does for writing what pauses do for speech. It is often better to break long sentences down into shorter ones than to worry about whether to use brackets or dashes. The importance of punctuation is shown in the following examples, which use the same words but mean completely different things:

'Teenagers, who drive carelessly, should not be allowed to have a driving licence.'

'Teenagers who drive carelessly should not be allowed to have a driving licence.'

The correct use of English

Unfortunately many people have not had the benefit of learning the rules of written English, even though we pay attention to such disciplines when we learn a foreign language. Consequently, by the time they come to study and work, they do not feel at ease with the demands of producing the wide range of written documents required of them. This section looks at some of the pitfalls.

Spelling

There are those who can and those who can't. If you have a spelling checker on your wordprocessor, make sure that it is appropriate for your work. That is, does it have English or American spelling – e.g. programme or program; centre or center?

Couples

Some words look and sound similar but cause confusion. Examples of such 'couples' include:

- principle/principal
- practise/practice
- stationery/stationary
- dependent/dependant
- complement/compliment.

Do you know the difference between them in all cases?

Similar words

There are other pairs of words that are similar in sound or spelling but which have distinct meanings. They include:

- practical/practicable
- disinterested/uninterested
- continual/continuous
- effect/affect.

Are you sure when these should be used?

Apostrophes

Apostrophes are used in two ways. The first use is to indicate that letters or figures have been omitted (e.g. It's for It is; or '95 for 1995). The second use is to indicate what is known as the 'possessive case' – that something belongs to a word or person (e.g. the book's pages = pages belonging to the book; or the child's toys = toys belonging to the child). Apostrophes should *not* be used to indicate plural as in 'hot drink's served here' or 'hundred's of jobs for temp's'.

- 'It's' means 'It is'. The apostrophe shows that something has been left out – in this case, the 'i' of 'is'. In 'What's your name?' it is the 'i' of 'What is your name?' that the apostrophe replaces.
- 'We have dealt with our parent's problems for many years.' Parent's = the problems of our (one) parent. Parents' = the problems of our (several) parents.

There is nothing to hide in finding writing difficult. It probably was not given the attention it deserved in college. Be honest with yourself and spend some time confronting the problem and practising the skill. You will be a more confident manager as a result.

Letter writing

As a manager you will have to write letters, and for most people this takes practice. Even if you do not have a natural flair for the written word, follow a few simple rules and your letters will be clear and present a good image of you and the work you do.

Prepare thoroughly

- Make sure that you are addressing the recipient of the letter in the correct way, or the way she/he prefers.
- Collect together the necessary support material, such as previous correspondence and relevant files, so you have to hand all the facts you need.
- Note down what you need to say in a logical order. At first you may have to write down most of the letter, but as you become more confident you will manage with a list of headings to remind you of what you want to say.
- Research the extra information you need such as unusual spellings of names, places or products, references, enclosures and extra copies. Also consider how you will address the recipient. Is he 'Dear Sir', 'Dear Mr Jackson', 'Dear David' or 'My Dear Dave'? The salutation may set the tone for the rest of the letter.

You are now ready to write the letter.

Identify the subject

The easiest way of referring to the reason for writing is to have a heading at the beginning of the body of the letter, as in the following example:

Dear Dave and Jill

CHANGE IN NURSERY HOURS

As you reminded me, . . .

If you have been in contact with the recipient before, it will be useful to summarise what has gone before. This is particularly important if there is any chance of misunderstanding, so that any potential problems may be identified quickly. You must be sure that your facts are accurate and that you present them clearly and concisely:

> *'As you reminded me, you contacted me following the parents' evening to discuss your requirement for Lucy's hours in the nursery to increase. I understand that you would like Lucy to attend on Thursdays as well as Tuesdays and Wednesdays, as from 1 March 1996.'*

You then let the recipient know what action needs to be taken and who will be responsible for it:

> *'We are pleased to be able to accommodate this, and I am enclosing an amended Parent/Nursery Contract for you to sign and return. This shows the fees that will be payable from 1 March.'*

You should end your letters with simple, polite statements that leave the reader feeling positive and not left hanging in mid-air:

> *'We look forward to seeing both you and Lucy more often in the nursery.'*

When you read through the finished letter, you should feel happy that it has set the right tone and is consistent with your relationship with the recipient. It should not be too familiar or too abrupt and, as well as covering all the facts, it should be easy to read.

4

Investing in People

- Professional Development

- Leader-generated Development

- The Investor in People Scheme

- A Career Development Model

- Delegating

- Recruiting Staff

- Appendices

Professional Development

'Learning' is not the province of the leader, the owner, the personnel function or the management group, it is the immediate responsibility of those to whom it happens. Personnel functions may well act as postroom for the organisation of training courses and the selection of appropriate developmental processes, but the learning itself is the province of individuals themselves, led by a *learning leader* – the nursery manager.

In order to retain good people for as long as possible, they need to be included, nurtured and developed and to keep learning with you. If this is done, you can honestly state that frequently abused term, 'people are our greatest asset'.

It is a current trend for managers to be held accountable as counsellors and coaches of their teams. Effective indications of success in this area are staff turnover, sickness levels and the rate at which staff develop.

The context for management and organisational development has changed. Thanks to the work of Charles Handy, John Constable and Roger McCormick, in the late 1980s, various issues have since led to the development of the Management Charter Initiative and the wealth of national competencies for all managers, through National Vocational Qualifications. For people in early years' services, management competencies will become apparent in NVQ level 4, yet to be developed. There are currently a variety of early childhood studies courses, ranging from NVQ level 2 through to postgraduate degrees (see Chapter 3). At undergraduate level courses do not usually provide an opportunity for in-depth study of the practical application of aspects of theory of early childhood development. Postgraduate courses are more often workplace-based, thereby offering an environment for those wishing to bring knowledge, skills and experience to bear on a pertinent problem within their professional situation, and to observe the effects over a substantial period of time. However, in the meantime, nursery managers are finding it worthwhile to explore NVQ assessor competencies, which provide qualifications to assess NVQ candidates in the workplace, and at the same time to acquire a useful management discipline of evaluation. The Management Charter Initiative (MCI) had led to the development of a Code of Conduct for Management Development (Figure 15) which amounts to a pledge, on the part of an organisation joining the MCI, to communicate and demonstrate the importance of management education and development.

This country also has extensive experience with 'distance learning packages', using radio and television and the postal system to deliver specific assignments, and tutorial support. The market covers informal short courses to fully approved university degrees.

A further move, most recently, has been in the development of an Individual Training Organisation (ITO) for the care sector (including childcare).

Another initiative, which is catching on fast, is the *Personal Development Agreement*. This is a contract between the individual and the organisation which states that, for a given output of

CODE OF CONDUCT

When your organisation joins the MCI, it makes a pledge to both current and future managers through the 10-point Code of Practice.

Chief Executives will communicate and demonstrate to all managers their commitment to this Code. It is a formal recognition of the importance of management education and development. Your organisation will promise:

1. To improve leadership and management skills throughout its structure.

2. To encourage managers continuously to develop their management and leadership skills.

3. To provide a coherent framework for self-development within the context of corporate goals.

4. To ensure that the development of managerial expertise is a continuous process, fully integrated with the work flow.

5. To provide ready access to relevant learning and development opportunities – both internal and external – with requisite support and time released, appropriate to the organisation.

6. To encourage and help managers acquire recognised relevant qualifications.

7. To participate actively in the appropriate MCI Networks.

8. Directly and through Networks, to strengthen links with management education sources, ensuring that the training offered will best complement management development programmes – matching corporate needs and future requirements.

9. To contribute to closer links with educational establishments.

10. To appoint a director or equivalent to oversee the fulfilment of these undertakings; to review progress annually and, after evaluating the contribution to performance, set new targets for both the individuals and the organisation; and to publicise highlights from the review and the new targets.

Figure 15. The Management Charter Initiative Code of Conduct.

work and the achievement of mutually agreed targets of performance and behaviour, the organisation will encourage activities of the individual to develop personally and, by extension, the organisation.

Note that it is a 'personal development' agreement, not a technical training one. It is about more than getting the job done, via the inclusion, competence and development route outlined in Chapter 1, and it has four aspects:

- personal development;
- professional development;
- team development;
- organisational development.

For each individual a time and money budget needs to be agreed. These details can be incorporated in a regular appraisal system. This facilitates a linking between personal needs and organisational targets. The personal development aspect can cover anything from physical fitness to studying for a part-time degree, the essence being personal challenge and growth.

This will be least influenced by organisational targets, and consequently is the most overlooked in terms of an activity that is seen as fruitful and worthwhile, altogether too soft for many managers. However, just as we believe, in our approach to children's learning, that care and education are inextricably linked, so we should be well placed to pursue achievement through nurturing, rather than accepting the more macho approach of bringing things under one's control and imposing one's will.

There is another reason why, once we realise it, we are in a good position to follow the people development path. Parents rate highly the continuity of nursery staff. It must therefore make commercial sense to bring on our own people, in whom we have *already made* the investment. If we do not, it diminishes the perceived worth of existing staff and de-energises them.

Leader-generated Development

This involves setting mutually agreed targets with individuals and teams, planning how to achieve them and delegating the authority to get on with it, and then monitoring the reality – the 'eyes on, hands off' approach. This can be as simple as the 'One Minute

Manager' notion of one minute's praise, one minute's criticism, per person, per day.

The basis of this approach lies in understanding that coaching is not teaching. It is not telling people what and how to do something, but getting them to develop a closer and closer focus on the way they do it – to question, monitor and give feedback.

A more nurturing and empathetic approach is to become available as a counsellor, putting oneself in the other's position and to start from where they are, rather than question the way they have gone about tackling the problem to date.

'Mentoring' is a further means of developing staff, more popular in the USA than here. Someone more senior is given responsibility to bring the individual on and to make best use of their contribution. The mentor is not the nursery manager or line manager and is generally concerned with wider issues than just performance in the job. There can, however, be problems when mentoring is formally established. Mentors can become patronising, or have their own motivations for being a mentor – perhaps wishing to muster support for a particular work method.

'Job rotation' is frequently overlooked as a low-cost means of extending the experience of staff and providing new challenges for those seeking promotion. It fits in with the concept of self-development, and complements inclusion and shared culture as fundamental aspects of investing in people.

The more traditional development and external training courses, although more expensive, can add a wholly different dimension to individual and organisational learning. Participants in open courses (i.e. those with no entry qualification required) rate their usefulness as:

- getting views and experiences of others in similar positions;
- getting views and experiences of those outside the industry;
- making contacts for future career possibilities;
- having a break from usual routine;
- gathering new knowledge, skills and techniques.

So, they generate different perspectives, encourage debate and broaden understanding. It is, however, questionable whether they contribute to performance and behaviour – the essence of competence.

Tailor-made, in-company courses, on the other hand, are gaining in favour. They can focus on key groups, on specific topics and be highly practical – allowing participants to return to their job and put something they have learned into practice immediately. At worst, as the facilitator or speaker will have been briefed by the organisation itself, they can reinforce existing prejudices and block change.

The Investor in People Scheme

This is a national scheme that encourages organisations to recognise the importance of developing staff to meet business objectives. The scheme recognises that every organisation is unique, just as every employee is an individual. But, in the same way, there are certain factors that are common to all. Organisations employ people and, whatever the business, the way those people perform will be a major factor in its success or failure.

People who are flexible and adaptable, who are willing to learn, and enthusiastic about the business and about their work, must be valuable assets in any organisation. Investor in People is based on the experiences of all types and sizes of successful UK companies that have proved that performance is improved by a planned approach to:

Setting and communicating business goals
Developing people to meet these goals

so that

What people can do and are motivated to do
Matches what the business needs them to do

Working towards meeting the Investor in People standard will in itself bring many benefits along the way, through the increased involvement and contribution of people at all levels within the organisation.

Being recognised as an Investor in People will increasingly be found to be of value, in the eyes of potential recruits as well as current employees, those with a stake in the business, and ultimately parents and suppliers.

An Investor in People improves individuals' performances by planning and taking action to improve the skills, knowledge, motivation, commitment, confidence and job satisfaction of all its people. Actions include developmental activities like:

- induction of new recruits;
- communications with employees;
- agreeing targets and standards for competence;
- encouraging attainment of appropriate qualifications and career progression;
- management development.

An Investor in People also takes action to ensure that all employees are aware of the contribution they can make to success – and that people then have the opportunity to make that contribution.

The national standard is a benchmark against which all organisations can measure their own commitment to and effectiveness in investing in people. The standard is founded on the four principles of commitment, planning, action and evaluation:

- *Commit* to investing in people to achieve business goals
- *Plan* how skill needs of individuals and teams are to be developed to achieve these goals
- *Act* to develop and use necessary skills in a well-defined and continuing programme
- *Evaluate* progress towards goals, value achieved and future needs.

Clearly it is possible to realise some benefits without going through the full Investor in People process, but the four principles of the standard interrelate. Working through them step by step will provide a focus and structure for your efforts. Once an organisation has been assessed as meeting the standard, it is publicly recognised as an Investor in People.

Many of the companies that have achieved the standard or who are working towards it are small or medium-sized businesses. In fact the process is more straightforward for smaller organisations with face-to-face communications and few tiers of management.

Becoming an Investor in People will need commitment and an investment of time, from you downwards. But it is not necessarily about doing more training or spending more money. It is about doing the training that is essential for the nursery and developing people more effectively to achieve your goals.

The actual cost will depend on what you do already, the

resources you have, how you match up to the national standard, and what you have to do to meet it. Your first priority will be to take charge of progress – or make someone in the company responsible for it – and put in enough time and resources to get things done.

Assessment and recognition of organisations is coordinated by Training and Enterprise Councils (TECs) in England and Wales and Local Enterprise Companies (LECs) in Scotland. Each TEC and LEC offers a range of services and support to help you become an Investor in People. You will work closely with the TEC or LEC throughout the process. Some of these services are free or subsidised for smaller businesses. Your local TEC or LEC will be pleased to discuss these with you.

Your local TEC or LEC has a set of action materials – a 'toolkit' – to help you through the process. They may be able to put you in touch with other organisations in your area who are working towards the standard. Talking to other small-business people may help you to see what sort of commitment you are taking on, what you need to do next and the benefits that come once you start.

First you must assess where you are now against the standard and the actions you will have to take. The toolkit includes a checklist, 'How do we measure up?'. Then you will need to produce an action plan with priorities, targets, resources and timescales. The accolade Investor in People cannot be achieved overnight: the time your organisation will take will depend on what has to be done and the resources you have available to do it.

The national standard for effective investment in people

An Investor in People makes a public commitment from the top to develop all employees to achieve its business objectives:

- Every employer should have a written but flexible plan which sets out business goals and targets, considers how employees will contribute to achieving the plan and specifies how development needs in particular will be assessed and met.
- Management should develop and communicate to all employees a vision of where the organisation is going and the contri-

bution employees will make to its success, involving employee representatives as appropriate.

An Investor in People regularly reviews the training and development needs of all employees:

- The resources for training and developing employees should be clearly identified in the business plan.
- Managers should be responsible for regularly agreeing training and development needs with each employee in the context of business objectives, setting targets and standards linked, where appropriate, to the achievement of National Vocational Qualifications (or relevant units) and, in Scotland, Scottish Vocational Qualifications.

An Investor in People takes action to train and develop individuals on recruitment and throughout their employment:

- Action should focus on the training needs of all new recruits and continually developing and improving the skills of existing employees.
- All employees should be encouraged to contribute to identifying and meeting their own job-related development needs.

An Investor in People evaluates the investment in training and development to assess achievement and improve future effectiveness:

- The investment, the competence and commitment of employees, and the use made of skills learned, should be reviewed at all levels against business goals and targets.
- The effectiveness of training and development should be reviewed at the top level and lead to renewed commitment and target setting.

A career development model

A career development model within a nursery setting could look like Figure 16.

This model does not imply that people can choose their jobs, but rather that the responsibility for putting themselves forward is theirs rather than just the manager's. If they are found to be ready to progress then they should be helped to prepare by the manager.

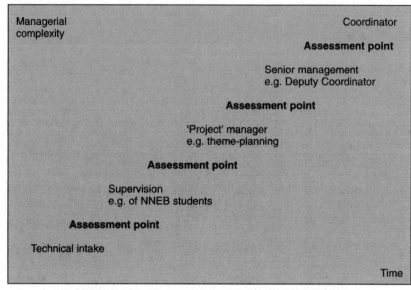

Figure 16. Nursery management career model.

If there is no higher job available to them, then they should be helped to broaden their experience whilst a suitable job is found.

To be effective and gain respect, an *appraisal system* must measure, debate and plan individual development and work targets, and generate useful feedback in both directions. It should:

- have a means of mutual discussion of past performance, present reality, and future opportunities and targets;
- relate to measurable work performance and target setting;
- focus on observable behaviour rather than speculation on hazy queries of personal qualities;
- relate directly to individual pay packages;
- draw out training and development needs and contract to action on them;
- show next possible career steps and why;
- give an overview of likely ultimate career stage;
- have a fair appeal system.

The essence of such a system is the individual's performance in their job. This may seem an unnecessary statement, but many appraisals are more to do with the manager's personal views of the individual's characteristics. That approach short-changes the individual and has led to cases of 'undue care' being cited as a claim against employers.

The appraisal should be completed in pencil by both appraisee and appraiser before they meet, at which point they should agree a mutual scoring and a plan. Most people underscore themselves and have to be coaxed into agreeing a higher score.

The most successful appraisal systems start with measurable *performance indicators* of past work. They state targets, quality, resource usage, illnesses, etc., agreed at the previous appraisal and measure them against present reality.

The rating of *behaviour* is also fundamental to the appraisal system. Behaviours are observable and can be easily checked out if there is disagreement. 'Behaviours' are not 'characteristics', such as honesty, integrity, etc., which are highly subjective; they are directly related to the aims and style of the organisation. If you need a creative, responsive, customer-friendly, nurturing type of organisation, a measurable behaviour might be 'is seen to work well in all areas of the nursery' or 'is able to form effective working relationships with all members of the team'. If you want a calm, methodical, judgemental type of organisation, you may consider that measurable behaviour such as 'is seen to make effective use of own/other people's time' is appropriate.

It has been found to be particularly powerful to involve staff in helping to agree the 'behaviours' for such a scheme. This has an energising effect and reinforces the shared culture of the organisation, as well as ensuring that people are committed to the appraisal process. The output from what are, typically, ten to twenty amenable behaviours can be plotted individually, and collectively, for feedback or trends in the organisation. In this way, the appraisal becomes part of *organisational learning*. The same behaviour with different targets should be capable of being used throughout the organisation.

From these measures of achievements and behaviours:

- new targets for the next period can be agreed;
- training and development needs can be identified and specified;
- next possible career steps can be discussed;
- concern about system/measurements can be taken forward, possibly to an identified 'external' appraiser.

There are several cost-effective ways of ensuring that personal development agreements are fulfilled. One is to use your staff as a training resource. Encourage staff to collect examples of details gone awry and to share their observations at an informal lunch. The informality should also strengthen ties between centrally based and 'field' staff.

Another way is to increase staff commitment to the firm by encouraging future senior staff to recruit new staff. This grants them a major responsibility while providing new staff with mentors who are not 'masters'.

Focus, too, on personnel relations. New members of staff should be greeted with a handbook of practice procedures, including basic information on management and administrations and quality-control expectations (see Chapter 2). Also, budget resources for educational activities. Every member of staff should be encouraged with a budget of time and money to take advantage of formal educational opportunities to maintain and develop existing skills. Encourage an awareness of new skills required, so that every member of staff is in a position to keep up to date with and initiate new ways of learning.

Delegating

It is absolutely clear that if you are trying to grow and develop the nursery, you will have more to communicate. Briefing groups are an excellent discipline for downward communication but there's a lot more to it than that. You need processes to ensure upward communication, and especially to coordinate across the organisation. So what is *your* best role and what must you look for in your deputy, administrative assistant, accountant, etc.?

Delegation – a remedy for overwork

Overwork is a common complaint of the small-business owner or manager: too much hard work and never enough hours in the day to do it. However, it is a problem that could easily be remedied by some effective delegation.

Delegation is simply the art of getting things done through other people. And if you show any of the following symptoms you should consider building delegating into the management of your business. Do you:

- have problems with deadlines for jobs that you do?
- have to work late regularly?
- take work home regularly?
- avoid accepting help with jobs?
- devote a lot of your time to details rather than planning and managing?
- feel insufficiently confident about your employees' ability to take on greater responsibility?

Delegation will help to keep the work flowing smoothly and so prevent a pile-up on your desk, which is both stress-inducing and counter-productive.

Fear of delegation

Most owner–managers are proud of the fact that they have built up their own company from nothing. In the beginning, entrepreneurs often perform all the tasks of running the business. This is reasonable enough, but as that operation grows they may hang on to too many jobs. They may believe that nobody else can do the job, and conversely it is just possible they may fear being shown up. It is also possible that, through pressure of work and the gradual nature of the expansion, they simply haven't reviewed the day-to-day management of their time.

Another reason for small-business owners not delegating is that sometimes the routine tasks are preferred to the difficult ones. Writing invoices is easier than preparing the new cash flow budget for the bank!

What has to be recognised is that when you delegate, both you and your employees get a chance to broaden skills. Through delegation you can ease your job of managing and thereby increase the effectiveness of both yourself and your workers – and thus your organisation.

Benefits for you

- *Delegation allows time to achieve more.* An owner–manager who can delegate effectively is likely to achieve greater output. Through the proper selection, assignment and coordination of tasks, a manager can mobilise resources to achieve more results than would have been possible without skilful delegation.

- *It allows time for managerial activities.* Delegation allows the owner–manager an opportunity to handle aspects of the job that no one else can do – project planning, plans for developing the business, monitoring how the business is doing, monitoring staff performance and dealing with any problems arising.
- *It provides you with back-up.* By delegating responsibility in different areas you will create a back-up workforce who can take over in times of emergency.

Benefits for staff

- *Delegation develops staff skills.* Owner–managers who fail to delegate effectively deprive staff of opportunities to improve their skills and assume greater responsibility. Since employees are likely to realise that they are not learning and gaining experience, they may well leave your firm in order to find a more challenging and supportive environment. This happens most frequently with those staff who are most talented – precisely the people you least want to lose. What is a routine job for you is often a growth opportunity for a member of staff.
- *It increases staff involvement.* Proper delegation encourages others to participate more in understanding and influencing their work. By increasing their involvement in the workplace you will also increase their enthusiasm and initiative for their work.

Benefits for your organisation

- *Delegation maximises efficient output.* It does this by making the best use of available human resources so as to achieve the highest possible rate of productivity. It also provides the right environment for staff to offer new ideas that can improve the flow and operation of the workplace.
- *It produces faster and more effective decisions.* An organisation is most responsive to changes in the environment when individuals closest to the problems are making the decisions about resolving those problems.
- *It increases flexibility of operations.* Effective delegation trains

several people to perform the same tasks. As a result, when someone is absent or when a crisis requires others to assist with functions not regularly a part of their job, several individuals will already be familiar with the assignment.

- *Delegation prepares people for promotion or rotation of responsibilities.* It also eases your job of finding someone to supervise when you are absent.

Your five-point plan

1. Decide what and what not to delegate

The general guidelines for deciding what should be delegated are:

- the work can be handled accurately by your staff;
- all necessary information for decision-making is available to the individual being delegated the task;
- the task involves operational detail rather than planning;
- the task does not require skills unique to the manager's position;
- an individual other than you has, or can have, direct control over the tasks.

Therefore any routine jobs of information collection, or assignments involving extensive detail such as making calculations, are things that can be delegated. Tasks that should *not* be delegated include the delegation process itself, employee appraisal and discipline, planning and forecasting, confidential tasks, complex situations and sensitive situations.

2. Decide to whom to delegate

Obviously your ability to delegate will be governed by the size and quality of your staff team at any given time. However, three factors are of primary importance when selecting the right person for an assignment: (a) their skills, (b) their interest, and (c) their workload.

3. Communicate your decision

Describe what it is you are delegating and give the other person enough information to carry out the task. Presenting the directive in writing will prevent the 'I didn't know' syndrome. If a gap exists between the assignment and an employee's skills you must be very clear and concise in describing the steps of the task.

Bear in mind that a new assignment, particularly one involving several stages, is unlikely to be completely understood on the first explanation. Make yourself available for further clarification as the staff member works through the assignment; close monitoring will save time in the long run.

4. Manage and evaluate

From the beginning, clearly establish set times when you will meet with the person to review their performance. The secret of delegation is to follow up.

5. Reward

Results that are recognised get repeated. You must monitor and respond to the person's performance. Otherwise it's like playing a game without keeping score, which in the end is not motivating.

Starting to delegate

Part of the essence of delegation is thoughtfully judging when a new employee is ready to handle a more stimulating assignment. If necessary delegate in stages, starting with small tasks and working up to more challenging projects.

Of course, the one thing you can never delegate is accountability. No matter who handles the task, as the manager it's your reputation that is on the line.

Delegation is a form of risk-taking, so if you cannot deal with a few mistakes you will never be able to delegate. Nonetheless, effective delegation that is carefully planned and well executed will result in a freeing-up of your time and a more efficient and more profitable business.

A summary checklist for effective delegation is included as an appendix to this chapter.

Recruiting Staff

Getting the right people is a difficult, time-consuming and costly business. Getting it wrong is even more expensive and can be extremely painful. Few growing businesses can claim not to have fallen into this trap. However, you can increase the odds on success by putting in place some basic processes and disciplines:

- Decide on the *numbers and skills mix* you are going to need over the next one to three years.
- Prepare *job descriptions* covering job titles and purpose, to whom responsible, limits of accountability and main tasks. A sample job description is included as an appendix to this chapter.
- Prepare a *person specification* outlining the sort of person you think is likely to be effective in the job.
- *Source your requirements creatively*, through networks of contacts, employment and search agencies, newspaper advertisements.
- *Weed out* application forms or CVs of those who don't fit the job description and person specification.

Forty-five seconds, it is claimed, is the time a typical manager takes from meeting an applicant before deciding whether or not he or she is the right person for the job. True or false, fears that the interview can be very subjective, and thus a biased way of selecting staff, are promoting the trend for companies to use standard measurement principles – such as those above – when recruiting.

Appendices to Chapter 4

Effective Delegation: A Synopsis

Principles

- Careful selection of jobs or assignments to delegate
- A clear view of the boundary between effective delegation and complete abdication
- Detailed planning and establishment of priorities
- Knowledge of delegate's capabilities, characteristics and experience
- Selection of proper delegate
- Establishment of goals and objectives for delegated tasks
- An understanding and agreement on standards of performance
- Provision for support as needed (volunteered and requested)
- Assessment of results and correction of errors
- Encouragement of independence
- Rewards or recognition where justified
- Acceptance by delegator of methods other than his/her own
- Establishment of trust and mutual understanding

Obstacles to delegation

- Inability of delegate to handle job (actual inability)
- Lack of confidence in delegate (perceived inability) in judgement, attitude, respect of others, etc.
- Fear of competition from delegate
- Exposure of weakness in delegator
- Lack of time for instructions and training
- Wish of delegator to do the particular job him/herself
- Belief by delegator that s/he is delegating adequately
- Perfectionism

Obstacles to acceptance of delegation by subordinate

- It is often easier to ask the boss than work it through
- Fear of criticism, especially when it is not fully warranted
- Lack of necessary information
- Lack of adequate resources
- Lack of self-confidence
- Lack of adequate incentive
- A feeling that the boss always wants his/her own way on what is done

Delegation usually works best when:

- delegate is physically distant
- delegator is absent frequently
- workloads are heavy
- there are many tight deadlines
- the organisation is young and vigorous with the emphasis on problem-solving
- standards of performance are attainable and fair
- the delegator feels personally secure
- a favourable environment exists which emphasises development, growth, innovation, creativity and human dignity
- a great deal of mutual trust exists at all levels of the organisation.

Job Description for a Nursery Officer

1.	POST:	Nursery Officer
2.	RESPONSIBLE TO:	The Nursery Coordinator, and in his/her absence the Deputy Coordinator
3.	OBJECTIVE:	To provide a high standard of daycare for children attending the nursery in accordance with company nursery management philosophy
4.	QUALIFICATIONS:	NNEB or equivalent with two years' post-qualification practical experience in daycare of the under-5s, preferably in a day nursery (some newly qualified candidates may be considered)

5. MAIN DUTIES

- To ensure that the children are cared for in a happy, safe and stimulating environment and to follow the principles of nursery management in the Company's Nursery Standards

- To have a sound understanding of a child's developmental needs and ensure these needs are met in an anti-racist environment

- To plan and provide a wide range of activities to meet the needs of all the children – both in groups and individually

- To maintain a high standard of hygiene and encourage the children to do the same

- To encourage the children to be independent and to learn to do things for themselves

- To be consistent and conduct him/herself in a professional manner at all times

- To abide by the policies of the nursery and put them into practice

- To cooperate and communicate with the Coordinator and Deputy Coordinator on nursery matters – both child and staff issues

- To work with and support other members of staff as part of a team

- To assist and supervise the training of students

- To participate in our inhouse training programme and take advantage of training courses made available

- To attend and contribute to staff meetings/parents meetings

- To liaise with parents and carers of children to whom they are the 'key worker' and discuss all matters relating to their child

- To liaise with outside agencies and sessional staff who visit the children in his/her immediate care, and to keep records of any treatment or therapy undertaken

- To pass on any relevant information to the Coordinator

- To carry out any domestic duties within the nursery as and when required.

5

Being an Ambassador

- Philosophy

- Philosophy Determines Priorities

- Promoting the Nursery

- Questions Parents Ask

- Working with Parents

- Networking

- Appendix

Philosophy

Angela Rumbold (1990) said that the aims of the curriculum will be most readily achieved where skilled and knowledgeable staff:

- have high expectancies of children; and
- value parents as their children's first educators and as active partners in the continuing process of education.

The involvement of parents in the care and education of their children is an important principle in the Children Act. The Social Services Inspectorate (SSI), in its inspection of private and voluntary day nurseries in 1995, found that the most common form of communication with parents was discussion at the times the children arrived and departed from the nursery. Parents confirmed their general level of satisfaction with this type and level of communication. The greatest satisfaction was obtained in nurseries where parents felt involved through regular meetings in discussion of their child's progress and care.

Is this really sufficient to engage the parent? Can they entirely appreciate the principles behind the way the nursery operates from this type of contact? The SSI went on to recommend that:

'*Consideration should be given to the use of contracts between nursery providers and purchasers of their services, that specify the quality of service to be provided.*'

There is no substitute for ensuring that, from the outset, parents understand through discussion and observation the underlying principles of care and education on which the service has been built. They form a reference point for future comment and contribution, without which parents' participation is often reduced to criticism. The SSI went on to say:

'*contracts ... that specified the quality of those services would provide a useful measure for parents ... to judge if the standards were met ...*'.

Although a manager must have backstops, a defence to depend on when faced with a complaint that should be entirely consistent with what has been described, he or she is primarily concerned that the situation does not reach the point of complaint. The ground needs to be covered at the outset.

Parents using a nursery will probably not be able to articulate the philosophy they seek, but they will recognise it when they see it in action, supported by having it described.

The pursuit of quality in education – and in particular in early childhood education – is high on the political and social agenda in the UK. A series of major national reports (Rumbold 1990; National Commission 1993, Sylva 1994) have argued strongly that educational provision for three- and four-year-olds should be expanded. Each report has also stressed the importance of high quality in this expansion and has specified in some detail what this should entail, at both a policy and practical level. The reports highlight the need for a national system of quality review and assurance and for a coordinated strategy of evaluation and development in early childhood settings.

This pressure for quality development flows alongside an acknowledgement of the valid and rigorously tested evidence that now exists showing that high-quality early childhood education can have a significant and long-term effect on children's learning, can lead to gains in educational achievement throughout schooling, and can lead to better social behaviour and more productive citizenship (Sylva 1994).

Young children in the UK are learning in a vast array of different settings, including local authority nurseries, primary schools, day nurseries, voluntary drop-in groups and playgroups, private kindergartens and workplace crèches and nurseries (see Figure 17). Each of these settings operates with different aims, funding, resources, staffing and quality-control procedures, and so the quality and effectiveness of the early-learning experiences they offer are variable. The result is that many of our young children do not receive the high-quality early-learning experiences they need to ensure a sound basis for later life.

In this context, provision for the under-fives in the UK remains patchy, diverse and – in comparison with other European countries – at a low level (Pascal 1990; Rumbold 1990; National Commission 1993; Moss 1994; Sylva 1994).

Parents' expectations of a nursery are likely to come from a list of things to look for which they have probably been given by a friend who has worked his or her way through the school system and has learned how to assess whether a school is right for their child.

- *Goldschmied and Jackson:* Working from what children can do (physical competence) and how they think. 'I can . . .', 'I know . . .'

- *Weikart* et al. *(High/Scope):* Children learning from real experiences and progressing to abstract signs; stages of representation through 'key experiences', towards understanding

- *Malaguzzi, Italy:* Towards communicating the 100 languages of children

- *Athey/Bruce/Nutbrown/Kellog:* Schema; threads of thinking; patterns of play; persistent cognitive concerns

- *Denmark (The Forest Nursery):* Learning in the open air; children learning about the natural world and using it for their play

- *Nurseryworks Ltd:* 'Workshop'; children as individuals with different needs, stages, learning patterns, interests

Figure 17.   Some examples of working models.

If a nursery follows a particular recognised vocational philosophy (e.g. Montessori, Steiner, Froebel) it may be reasonably straightforward to articulate, and parents will recognise what you are talking about. However, most do not, because their starting point is *not* that of a school but of a new provision – the dedicated under-fives provision for parents who have a choice. It is more likely that the nursery has drawn on a number of sources and developed a hybrid philosophy (see Figure 17).

What you can be certain of in the private sector is that it, the establishment, will have a philosophy – this is its marketing offer. And what is most essential to the owner of the nursery is that each and every staff member should ooze it. Very few parents will choose a nursery unseen, or on its literature alone.

Parents are the market. Nursery staff are ambassadors for the service in reaching that market. The perspective of parents is the external rationale for nursery nurses to appreciate the philosophy and approach of the setting they work in. But there are internal reasons as well.

Philosophy Determines Priorities

Some nurseries may be concerned with the order and pace of the day: everyone knowing what is expected of them and when; how long institutional functions should take; and how many activities and of what variety should take place each day. Others may consider that if a group of children is enjoying a particular activity, it doesn't matter that they are 'late' for tea.

All will have invested resources carefully, and it may be that the smooth running of the nursery relies on each activity being properly cleared away before the next one starts. Is it OK then, within the team, for one person to be allocated to sit and play with the expectant children, or should everyone be involved in clearing up so that everyone can move on together?

Harmony in the team is built on shared philosophies, mutual understanding and respect for why things are run as they are. In order to join the team, the nursery nurse must establish what he or she needs to know *before* starting, on the *first day* and during the *first few weeks*.

Before starting

'How is the nursery explained to parents?', 'Can I sign up to the philosophies as they are expressed?', 'Can I accept that the way we do things is . . . ?'

Being a manager means being able to share and promote the aspirations of the organisation, both internally and externally. Before taking on the role, it is important that you know where you stand on, for example, group care as distinct from one-to-one attention; babies in nurseries; the length of the nursery day; discipline of young children; taking young children into the workplace; the difference between a nursery, a nursery school, a playgroup, etc. It is reasonable that both staff and parents rely on you as a manager to articulate the philosophy of the organisation and believe it! Parents, particularly first-time parents, are anxious about all these issues, possibly do not know where they stand on many of them, and require constant reassurance that they are not leading their child along the wrong path.

It is equally important that staff can accept the way in which the nursery's philosophy is articulated to children: 'The way we behave towards each other in nursery is . . .'. This will usually involve a particular approach to equal opportunities, to the format and flow of the nursery day, and to the extent to which children of differing ages are grouped together. How strongly do you feel that, despite the cultural background of the child which may suggest a different approach in nursery, mealtimes are relaxed, social occasions? Or, how important is it that all children have the opportunity to access all core areas of activity every day? To what extent should four-year-olds be protected from the boisterous toddlers?

How familiar can staff be with parents? Who speaks to them about what? At what point is a member of staff expected to intervene in a child's activity? These are just some of the crucial things to get right on your first day as a manager, which means that you need to explore them before you begin.

It is important to know how the hierarchy and roles within the staff team work, and how each individual can influence the quality of service. Equally important is to know how the pattern might be upset. This is discussed in Chapter 4.

The first few weeks

Increasingly, you will be expected to explain and discuss with parents the nursery's viewpoint on all the foregoing issues. The areas for misunderstanding on the part of parents are numerous, and this – coupled with the level of detail about which parents expect to be informed – requires scrupulous attention to consistency on the part of staff. It is neither helpful nor fair to parents to have two differing versions of, for example, the nursery's discipline policy.

On their first visit, parents will want to see and feel:

- a welcoming atmosphere;
- children taking positive pride in their work and play;
- positive relationships between staff/children, children/children, staff/staff;
- positive documentation – what is being achieved;
- positive autonomy of staff – staff empowered and supported to make the appropriate decisions;
- positive awareness of the manager, and your familiarity with all current issues in the nursery;
- positive planning of activities – evidence that staff are proactive and take a real interest in the construction of a current programme for the children;
- positive expectations of children.

- Purposeful leadership
- Involvement of all staff in management
- Consistency of approach and methods amongst staff
- Planned and purposeful sessions
- Challenging teaching
- Work-centred environments
- Children's opportunity for debate
- Maximum communication between children and adults
- Up-to-date record-keeping
- Parental involvement
- Positive approach to improvement/development

Figure 18.   Factors critical to the effectiveness of a nursery.

The Inner London Education Authority *Junior School Project* (1980) identified that parents looked for signs, when visiting nurseries and primary schools, that would lead to their children:

'doing as well as possible'
'being happy and enjoying it'
'learning to be polite and well-behaved'
'reading and writing as soon as possible'.

Being an effective ambassador for the nursery is about describing the features of the nursery service in terms that parents can understand, appreciate and desire. Even though the academic underpinning for the service, and the motivation of the 'driving force', is probably why you took on the job, it is the translation of these into real benefits for the parents that will achieve your real goal – a full and thriving nursery. This translation process is detailed in Chapter 6. However, it is worth pausing here to consider the factors that have been found to be critical in achieving the outcomes for parents identified above (see Figure 18). They provide an agenda for review by the new manager.

Promoting the Nursery

Promotion is a catch-all word for marketing communications: advertising, personal selling, sales promotions and public relations. Doing business without promotion, it has been said, is like working in the dark: you know what you are doing but no one else does!

But promotion is probably the most intangible area of expenditure in a nursery business. Discovering exactly what benefits you get from the money you spend is a problem that taxes most business people. Lord Leverhulme, the founder of the soaps and detergents empire Lever Brothers, is reputed to have said 'I know half the money I spend on advertising is wasted. The problem is to know which half.'

Budgets are always tight in nurseries. If there is anything to spare, of course you want to spend it on improving the service – something of direct benefit to the children. A method of advertising needs to be chosen which you will get through to most of your likely parent group at least cost. Remember also that you do not generate bookings directly from advertising; it simply initiates that process, raises awareness of your particular service in the selected market. Bookings are made only once the advertising has taken effect and parents come to visit. There are a number of issues to be decided.

Segmenting the market: Who are you trying to attract?

What type of parent is going to share your interests and aspirations for young children, and where are they located? Do they belong to identifiable socio-economic groups, or do they need to, in terms of your fee structure? Your advertising choices must follow from the answers to these questions. Are you just looking to fill the nursery from your immediate local area, or is it a central point that parents pass through – on their way to work, for instance? Should you also then be looking at where they come from?

Setting advertising objectives: What are you asking parents to do?

Do you want them to ring you, visit the nursery, think again about nurseries versus nannies? The message must convey the response you expect the parents to make. You may believe that what you want to do is raise awareness of how your nursery differs from others, in the hope that parents will retain the message until they need to *use* the information. On the other hand, you may be issuing an invitation to visit the nursery for a specific purpose. It is useful to pinpoint precisely what is intended. Do you want to:

• increase telephone enquiries by say 10% over 6 months?

- raise awareness of the nursery in a previously untargeted residential area?
- generate an additional (say) 20 visits to the nursery before Christmas?

Defining the advertising message: What should you say?

Look at the nursery service from the parents' standpoint and answer the hypothetical question, 'Why should I book a place in your nursery?' It is best to consider the answer in two stages:

- 'Why should I book a place in *any* nursery?' What benefits will nursery care have over, say, nanny, childminder, or a nursery class?
- 'Why should I book a place in *your* nursery?' What advantages does your nursery have for me, over others?

From a parent survey we undertook in 1994 (see Chapter 7) we learnt a great deal about parents' priorities and aspirations for nursery care, and we have been able to incorporate these into our more recent advertising messages. Having said all that, the most effective form of advertising is the kind that existing parents do for you, by recommending your service to friends. Staying in touch with your present parents' wishes is a large element of your advertising plan, because it provides you with the information for what *they* want to hear, and pass on.

Deciding on the creative angle: How do we deliver the message?

Possibly the most important point to remember here is that you should not choose the medium *you* like best, but the one that is most appropriate (see Figure 19).

Not all methods of communication carry an equal impact. It has already been noted that by far the most effective form of advertising is that of a recommendation of a trusted friend. Here is a summary of the best uses of various other forms:

- Leaflets give a short, memorable, personal message.
- Newspapers can deliver longer, more complex, one-off messages.
- Magazines deliver highly targeted, complex messages.
- Radio and television convey short repeated messages.
- Outdoor billboards carry short, high-impact messages.

Straight facts	Yellow pages, Thomsons, etc.
Reasoning	Advert or article logically explaining the benefits of the nursery
Emotions	Advert associating the nursery with pleasant connotations or mood, or peace of mind
Hard sell	Advert commands action: 'Nurseries are good for you'
Endorsement	Advert uses role models: 'Snow White uses our nursery'

Figure 19. Choosing the medium for promotion.

- Indoor billboards carry more detailed, subtle messages.
- Transport interiors can have long, complex messages.
- Transport exteriors carry short, high-impact messages.

Setting the advertising budget: How much should you spend?

The 'What can we afford?' approach implies that advertising is an extravagance. Given what we know about the effects of occupancy levels on all aspects of service, this approach must be questioned.

A more logical approach is to look at how much you have been spending, and relate it to how you feel about occupancy. That is, if you spent 5% of total income last year and you are maintaining occupancy levels as intended, then there is little reason to suppose it needs changing.

The cost/benefit approach takes this one step further. If you reckon that a £250 advertisement 'cost' will generate 25 enquiries, and you know that 10% of enquiries generally turn into bookings, and you have the staffing, etc. in place to accept the additional children, in this case 2.5, then the 'benefit' to you is the profit margin on 2.5 places. This will provide you with some guidance on whether a particular advertising cost is worthwhile.

Measuring the results

Because advertising is expensive it is important to monitor the results of everything you do, and not to repeat wasted effort. Figure 20 shows how this could be done.

Such an analysis will help you to understand not only what enquiries are most likely to turn into bookings, but also how relatively expensive different forms of advertising are, and which are better used for raising general awareness of the nursery, and which for immediate bookings.

What exactly are you selling?

Having attracted parents to visit the nursery, how do you ensure that they collect all the information they need to make a decision to book a place?

A *passive* approach would be to describe what goes on in each area of the nursery, and allow the parent to take in as much as they could about nursery life.

A more *proactive* approach would be to consider what it is that your nursery offers over and above other nurseries, and to find a way of ensuring that the parent leaves in full knowledge of the benefits these features bring.

	LOCAL NEWSPAPER	LEAFLETS	POSTERS	PERSONAL RECOMMENDATION	TOTAL
Cost	£200	£100	£1000	£0	£1300
Telephone enquiries	50	30	100	10	190
Cost per enquiry	£4	£3.33	£10	£0	£6.84
Visits	5	20	20	10	55
Cost per visit	£40	£5	£50	£0	£23.64
Bookings	2	5	3	5	15
Cost per booking	£100	£20	£333	£0	£86.67

Figure 20. Measuring the results of advertising.

What are the components of the sales package? Firstly, the *service* itself:

- what it does and what it consists of;
- what children get out of it;
- what parents get out of it.

The way the service is described will be informed by what you know about the needs and aspirations of parents, and what knowledge and views you have on the way children develop.

It is important that the service be described in a way that the parent can understand. For example, if you have an organisational structure in which a group of children pursue individual academic goals through collaborative efforts, why not say that:

> *'Children learn and play in small groups around an activity that they have chosen.'*

What you think makes the nursery special may actually be meaningless to the parent who is rarely an early years' specialist, and it needs to be *translated* (see Figure 21). For instance, the staff ratio may be higher in your nursery than in others, or your staff team may be better qualified. You can deduce from this that your service is above average in quality, but saying that does not really do anything for the parent. If, however, the parent can see these aspects of your service as contributing to a better educational start for their child, then the message has been received.

FEATURES	BENEFITS TO CHILD	PARENTS' IMPRESSION
Above-average quality of service	Best start in life for child	Good parenting decision
Professional management	Reliable and financially stable	Value for money
Constantly developing/ innovative on service	Adapting to child's and parents' changing and individual needs	State-of-the-art purchase

Figure 21. Examples of translating features into benefits.

Questions Parents Ask

In my experience, there are a number of concerns that parents express, time and time again. The following represents a selection of answers that may be helpful.

'Why choose the nursery option? How can group care ever be better than the one-to-one attention of a nanny or childminder?'

Answer: 'Practically speaking, nurseries provide continuity. Nurseries don't get ill, go on holiday or hand in their notice. More important is the child's emotional stability. If a child is intensely attached to a single carer and that person then leaves for whatever reason, the experience can be deeply traumatic. Multiply that experience a few times and a child may become wary of making any attachments at all.

'A related issue is the jealousy and emotional conflict that some parents feel if their child becomes deeply devoted to the nanny to the exclusion of themselves. Our nurseries provide a dependable, secure environment which complements rather than supplants the parents' role. The confidence children acquire at nursery is broad-based, not contingent on a single relationship.

'The positive benefits of nursery care are far-reaching. By engaging in a group, children learn to respect others, to be aware of each others' needs, to share, take turns and cooperate in creative play and activity. All of these skills help to foster the development of language and communication, as children learn to interact with each other and those who look after them.

'A good nursery meets objective, measurable standards. Parents can see the quality of care that is offered and trust their choice to a far greater extent than if they were placing their child in the hands of just one person.'

'What about babies? Should babies be cared for in nurseries at all?'

Answer: 'Babies can and do flourish in a nursery environment, provided certain conditions are met. Babies have the ability to develop attachments with several people, but not with many people. For this reason, we take care to select and keep staff with the maturity and instinctive warmth to form close bonds with small babies and their parents – carers who are able to put the needs of babies first and follow their lead when it comes to play, activity and routine.

'The areas within nurseries specifically designed for babies offer calm, peaceful and stimulating surroundings where they can begin to explore the world.

'We know parents want their babies to be the focus of loving attention and this is what we provide.'

What is your attitude to discipline?

Answer: 'Recent research shows that this issue is of particular concern to parents of toddlers! This isn't surprising, since the toddler's desire for independence, knowledge and control over their world can often clash with the fact that they are still largely dependent on adults to make things happen.

'Confining children within a rigid set of imposed rules does little to foster true self-control. Our staff expect the best – not the worst – of the children in our care. Good manners, sociable behaviour, fairness and kindness all stem from a basic awareness of the needs of others, and every two-year-old needs support and encouragement to take this huge conceptual step. By promoting the core values of respect and self-esteem, sharing and participation, the nursery worker can guide the child through this challenging phase of development.

'Of course, behaviour that is harmful to the child or to others can never be tolerated or accepted. But understanding the reason for a tantrum or temperamental outburst, talking it through calmly with the child, proposing alternatives, are all part of the process of helping the child gain a better command of their emotions and show a positive response to others.'

'What provision do you make for pre-school children? Wouldn't this age group be better served by a nursery school?'

Answer: 'There is a clear distinction between day-centres – which are essentially focused on physical and emotional care – and nursery schools, either privately run or administered by education authorities – which are largely geared towards pre-school learning. What we aim to offer is 'educare', in the rather ungainly contemporary term, combining a nurturing and emotionally stable base with the opportunity to explore and develop new skills.

'We strongly believe that one cannot exist without the other; for young children these two aspects must be interdependent and intertwined. At our nurseries, you will not find a replica of a classroom environment with formal instruction in reading, writing, or arithmetic, or a simple minding service from nine to five. What you will find is an emphasis on "learning through living" and "learning through play". Our educational provision is not haphazard or unplanned, but based on a structured programme designed to engage children of different ages and levels of skill. A themed topic, for example 'autumn', can encompass a nature walk; the counting of leaves, acorns and conkers; a recognition of colour, texture and shape; seasonal stories, rhymes and songs; drawing and labelling.

'Through these varied and challenging means many of the children in our nurseries attain the standards laid down by the National Curriculum for primary schools – and, more importantly, have fun along the way.'

'Your nursery is located in the City. What can young children gain by accompanying their parents to work?'

Answer: 'Time is precious to working parents. Bringing children into the City, close to where you work, can make good use of what would otherwise be empty commuting time. Travelling in by train, bus or car offers the opportunity to share stories, songs – or just talk. A nursery near your office means you are close at hand – to share lunch with your child, join in birthday celebrations and activities – fathers, too! You are also nearby in the case of illness, or if extra demands at work disrupt your normal schedule.

'The City nursery provides all the resources of home-based care – libraries, swimming pools, parks and shops – with the important advantage that your child is included within the framework of your working world.'

'Your nurseries are relatively expensive. Isn't there any way of cutting costs?'

Answer: 'The short answer is no. We are dedicated to quality, surpassing the high standards laid down in legislation in every field – safety, educational provision, diet, outside activity and the design and equipping of our nursery spaces. But the highest proportion of our overhead goes on staff. There is no way of trimming costs without compromising our central philosophy, the nursery worker–child ratio, the level of dedication, effort and continuity we expect and achieve from those we employ.'

'How does nursery care benefit children in the long term? Is it the best start in life?'

Answer: 'Many studies suggest that nursery experience gives the child a flying start. Children who have been exposed to a wider social group and mix at an early age are generally better equipped to work in a team, to cooperate and share, and form good friendships and working partnerships during their years of formal schooling. Evidence suggests that they also go on to do better in terms of educational achievement, in the acquisition of reading, writing and numerical skills.

'All parents want the best for their children, and all parents want their children to achieve. But the desire for children to progress and perform must never be gained at the expense of their emotional needs. A child is only a child once. We believe in helping children realise their potential within a secure framework of care and support. The best start you can give your children is measured not only by their future prowess but in the quality of their daily experience now, in their present happiness, well-being and zest for life. This, essentially, is what we mean by putting the child first.

'At our nursery we respond to children. We take care to promote physical well-being, to stimulate development of new skills and to meet emotional needs.

'Teamwork is the cornerstone of our policy. We take care to select the best staff – to choose those who are bright, aware and enthusiastic – to build a community committed to the support of both parents and children.

'Children deserve the best environment to flourish and play in safety. We take care to design spaces that children enjoy, to equip and maintain our nurseries to the highest standard, to build in opportunities for exploration and discovery – to make children feel at home.

'A good environment also means stable routines and core values. We take care to balance activity with nurture, to foster sharing and participation, to encourage social interplay and individual expression, to build confidence and promote self-esteem.

'The early years represent a most intense period of growth and development in a child's life. Our expertise is founded on interaction with parents and children, thorough appraisal of the latest developments in educational thinking, and constant re-evaluation of needs and aims. We put your children first – because you do.'

Parents will also require more specific information about aspects of the nursery service. You must decide what your service priorities are. Here I offer my own, as a starting point.

Quality of care

The key-worker system

'Each child is assigned a key-worker with personal responsibility for overseeing progress and maintaining continuity. Children need a focus, a special person to whom to relate. Our key-worker system provides a dependable relationship to ease times of transition at the beginning and end of the day.'

Feedback

'Our staff are trained to make detailed observations of your child's progress. Friendly and responsive, they will always make time to share details of your child's daily achievements and activities, and respond to your concerns. Children delight in displaying their triumphs, from messing about with paint to using the potty unaided. Noticeboards provide an essential backup, displaying artwork, menus, news and information about activities.'

Environment

'Our nurseries have been specifically designed and equipped to provide a stimulating, child-centred environment which combines the friendly atmosphere of home with the opportunities to explore and widen experience.'

Food

'Mealtimes are important moments in the day. All meals are freshly prepared and cooked on the premises, taking into account specific cultural and dietary needs. Staff and children sit down together to eat in small family groups.'

Rest

'We ensure activity is balanced with regular periods of rest. Routine naps, periods of quiet activity and shared stories mean the child is not overtired, fretful or anxious at the end of the day. Variety of experience makes children eager to learn, while a familiar framework of orderly routines shapes the day and provides stability.'

Safety

'All our nurseries are regularly inspected and surpass the exacting standards required by current legislation. Our staff are fully trained in emergency and first aid procedures.'

Learning together

Following the child

'The open-plan nursery layout is organised to provide different centres of activity from which each child is free to choose. We believe in following and supporting the child's focus of interest, and respecting their choices, not directing or enforcing attention. Children may be invited to participate in shared activities, but never compelled.'

Exploration and discovery

'Children investigate the world through all the senses – touch, taste, smell, sight and sound – and in the process discover exciting new concepts – heavy and light, before and after, high and low. By broadening the realm of experience we provide the opportunity to explore and experiment. To a child, an educational toy can be a bunch of keys, a sponge, a ball of wool, a funny hat, a bucket of sand, a string of beads – everyday items that can serve as vehicles for the acquisition of new manipulative and cognitive skills.'

Stages

'Babies start by exploring you and themselves, then greedily seize the world of colour and shape and texture, learning through focused attention and observation. Toddlers love to copy and mimic and need role models for their boisterous activity. Through dismantling and constructing they test the limits of their world and begin to learn independence. Pre-school children are ready to share and respond to the challenge of teamwork and activities that extend their concentration. Our child-centred programmes are designed to respond to each child individually and support their own path of development.'

Structured programme

'The role of the nursery worker is to facilitate learning experience, to engage with the child and support emerging skills and interests. It looks like play – and it is – play with a purpose. We offer a wealth of different activities to provide a fresh and challenging environment for discovery and fun. Each activity is planned to ensure it offers the potential to challenge children at different levels of development.'

Language

'Language is the key to learning. Names and labels, songs, stories and rhymes promote literacy and verbal fluency. Group care brings wider exposure to language and fosters communication skills.'

Consultation

'Our nursery programmes are the result of a constant process of refinement and development. Consultation with childcare and education professionals informs our thinking and practice. Just as important, we listen to parents to find out what they want for their children. Regular get-togethers enable everyone to share their views and initiate new approaches.'

Terms and conditions

The second part of what you are selling is the contract to which you are asking parents to commit. It is vital that parents read and understand the essential points before they book a place. Do not underestimate the damage that can be done to relations with parents, quite apart from the business, of terms and conditions of contract not being properly understood.

Of course, the last thing parents want to hear when they are delighted to have found your nursery, and decide to book a place, are the rather negative-sounding messages contained in 'notice periods' and 'deposits'. However, there is no substitute for being crystal clear about these issues from the outset. In particular, make sure that parents understand the following:

- deposit arrangements;
- fees;
- payment terms;
- notice of withdrawal period.

The appendix to this chapter contains specimen 'terms and conditions'.

Showing parents round the nursery

Start with what the parent already knows about nurseries in general, and your nursery, in order that you are not using up precious time repeating what they know. Also, find out from the parent where their main concerns lie. Is it returning to work or leaving their child, or safety aspects, or education? This will provide you with a framework for showing the parent the nursery, for pausing in the right places, for relevant introductions to other staff.

We have found that encouraging parents to spend time with staff in the area that currently interests them most (e.g. the baby unit) provides them with lasting insights into nursery life and gives them much confidence at a time when they are feeling vulnerable in a nursery setting. It is also important for parents to have a feel for the character and competence of staff other than yourself, as it is unlikely that you will actually have intimate care of their child.

Working with Parents

Combining work and family

The majority of parents who choose to use private nurseries are working. This is because very often a private nursery is the only group provision available to them, but also this form of provision has become popular with working parents because its focus is on providing a service that is flexible to their needs as well as reflecting their aspirations for their child.

However, whereas five or six years ago most of the demand was for full-time places, and part-time usage was considered as a secondary market by those who started nurseries, it would be ignored at the nursery's peril today. Several aspects of family and working life have converged to make part-time provision more attractive:

- The 1990s have brought a greater concern for well-being, a grave concern about the level of stress that working parents were bringing on themselves during the period of exceptional economic activity in the 1980s.
- The quality of their own and their child's early experiences are current and newsworthy issues, which has led to a greater awareness of what constitutes 'quality' and a parallel expectation of any childcare service, and the attendant high cost.
- Employers are less interested in providing childcare themselves as a remuneration 'benefit', preferring to support the employee's own arrangements as a reflection of a human resources family-friendly attitude.

All this has focused the minds of those parents who wish to combine a career with bringing up a family on the relationship between quality and cost. There is a trend towards opting for part-time provision rather than accepting a compromise, on their own or their child's behalf, for the sake of a full-time place.

A major source of anxiety for parents is how to combine work and parenthood (Katz 1994). Even now the majority of parents rely on an informal network of friends and family to provide childcare, which may include one parent providing the care whilst the other parent works (Cohen 1990). In the absence of subsidy, the cost of full-time private childcare – which is where the widest expansion of services has been in the last decade – is still prohibitive to many. As a proportion of the total number of children of working parents, the number in nurseries remains very low. Against this background, whereas childminding provided by both relations and childminders (a one-to-one form of childcare) represents the most widely used provision, it is likely that parents using a nursery will not necessarily be accustomed to participating in a community when it comes to the care of their young child.

Further, parents are mindful that in the UK we are still debating the benefits to the child and to the parent, of both parents working. Leach (1994), for example, states:

'*Babies and young children have to be cared for by committed adults in suitable environments for 24 hours of every day. Society expects all able-bodied citizens of working age to earn the money they need and the satisfaction they crave at specialised all-day jobs in special, distant and unsuitable places. People cannot be in two places at once; ergo one person cannot be simultaneously a solvent, self-respecting citizen and an actively caring adult.*'

However, Bettleheim (1987) argues:

'*In order to raise a child well one ought not to try to be a perfect parent, as much as one should not expect one's child to be, or to become, a perfect individual. Perfection is not within the grasp of ordinary human beings. Efforts to attain it typically interfere with that lenient response to the imperfection of others, including those of one's child, which alone make good human relationships possible.*'

In their research into childcare information services, Hogg and Harker (1992) pointed out that:

'*[A workforce] is comprised of individuals with full and complex lives outside the workplace. A family-friendly employer asks employees about their experiences and involves them in forming and implementing policies through effective communication and training.*'

So, too, should parents be involved in the development of the nursery. The contribution of parents begins with familiarity with the nursery service and this process can be started when the first visit takes place. Parents should understand that from this point on they will be included in service arrangements, and that they will, it is hoped, never be taken aback by a situation that arises. This is not only about ensuring that parents are fully informed of developments concerning their child; good atmosphere is dependent on the participation of the whole community coming in and out of the nursery, and policies need to be devised that positively promote the involvement of parents in the development of the nursery itself and encourage a partnership concept of shared care.

Nursery and parents as partners

There is no substitute for giving parents the opportunity to experience at first hand how their children will spend their day and the benefits that the nursery environment will bring to the children. As much time as possible should be afforded to the parents to enable them to feel happy and positive about the nursery environment, and to ensure that they are introduced to each aspect of the nursery service. We have found that, should a problem arise at a later date, it can invariably be traced back to the parent not having been made aware of that particular procedure or approach, either because the settling was rushed or for the lack of opportunity to experience nursery life.

Working parents are a transitory population and turnover of parents in the nursery will be high. This means that, although it is important for parents to have an overview of the whole service offered by the nursery, it is equally important that they be reminded of the next phase of the service as their child prepares for it. If they join when their child is a baby then their greatest concerns and interest will be with the baby unit, its staff and routines. Although parents will acknowledge and hear your explanation of the changes in the curriculum as a child develops and grows, they will probably not be so questioning as those who are entering their child at two years. So, settling is not just a once-off process; it must be followed up and parents resettled at each phase-change.

It should now be regarded as normal practice in nurseries for parents to be welcomed into the nursery at any time of day, to observe or to take part in activities with their child and others. Working parents frequently find themselves precluded from this because of the pattern of their working day, so that contact is limited to arrival and collection times. Interestingly, although we have critics of our nursery in the City of London from the point of view of commuting with young children, we experience more daytime visits from parents there than at any other of our nurseries, because we are adjacent to the workplace. However, the nursery is independent (i.e. it is not attached to any one company's workplace), and so there is no concern on the part of the parents that they should not be seen to be there during the day, because they should be 'at work'. It is also worth noting that the nursery has provided an unusual opportunity for fathers to involve themselves in playing with their baby and feeding, when in almost any other circumstances they would be denied this chance while they are commuting to work in a metropolitan area.

In our nurseries we actively encourage parents to get involved in story-telling and outings with other children as well as their own. If they have any special talents, such as playing a musical instrument, dancing or pottery, they are encouraged to come in and take small groups of children together with a member of staff. A Parents' Notice Board displays items of current interest from the press or local events, and requests for special resources – in particular, items from other cultures and countries to support a curricular theme. Daily diary displays illustrate what has been going on in nursery that day, and individualised charts provide a flavour of how each child's day has been spent. This includes not only essential information about meals, naps and changes, but also the activities in which they were most engaged and who they played and worked with.

Rounding-off-the-day discussions are encouraged. This time is used for following up on the observations made by staff, which will contribute to the child's profile records. This is particularly important for babies as they are non-verbal and develop dramatically in short spaces of time. The sharing of information enables staff and parents to be more aware of the new skills their baby is acquiring and provide more focused attention to their current needs.

Organised parents' sessions are usually welcomed, but for busy people such events need to respond to a real need on the part of the parents or the nursery, so that time can be set aside to attend. We have found that occasional social events with staff are popular. However, parents network anyway and many longlasting friendships between parents have been founded in the nursery quite informally. We have also found that parents welcome information about child development and help with the choices they must make as their child grows. The most successful parents' sessions we have held have been where an expert speaker has led discussion on an identified parental concern, such as choosing a school, early childhood illnesses and early literacy. Such events provide the nursery with the added opportunity to remind parents of nursery policy as well as to hear current parents' views.

Steering groups

Many nurseries have Steering Groups or Consultation Groups which are used as a forum for reviewing policy and contributing new ideas. These usually meet regularly throughout the year and can be a very important means of ensuring that the nursery does not become an island, limited by its own daily experiences. The membership of such a Group needs to be carefully considered alongside the Group's purpose or remit. In particular, it is important that the terms of reference of the Group are well understood and agreed in order that expectations of members are in line with the way the nursery intends to act on the discussion held. Although we are not required to have a Group in our nurseries, which are independent, we find them invaluable for informing us of local initiatives that may otherwise go unnoticed and for widening our thinking about the expectations of parents and entitlements of children. These being our purposes, membership of our Groups reflects this and includes parent representatives, a local primary headteacher, a tutor from the local NNEB college, and a community representative, as well as corporate clients. This last group is essential if the nursery is used as a workplace nursery within the Inland Revenue's definition.

All these different ways of communicating with parents, and encouragements to working as partners in the care and education of their young children, help us to reassure parents of the benefits of using a nursery, and remind them of our policies on the difficult issues of managing children's behaviour and dealing with childhood illnesses. They also help us to keep in touch with parents' changing needs and aspirations.

Networking

A nursery can benefit a great deal from being part of the community it serves. This sounds obvious, but it is frequently not the case because of the way in which it came into being or because of where it is located. If the nursery is to benefit, its relationship with the community needs to go further than the formal liaison with other professionals required under the Children Act provisions which protect the welfare and health of the child.

Community links

As part of the nursery curriculum children will visit local libraries, swimming pools, parks, and other resources that add richness to daily activities. They also have the opportunity to do things they would be doing if they were with their parents, such as shopping and going for walks. Ideally the nursery children will visit schools and be invited to watch special shows and assemblies to introduce them to school life. All this activity can help to broaden the children's perspective and encourage them to explore places and people in a positive way.

However, this can be a two-way process, with the nursery offering some of its resources to others in the community. School children can be invited to observe some of the nursery routines; and nursery dancing and music classes can be extended to children in the care of local childminders – also providing an opportunity for the carers to get to know the nursery staff. Holiday playschemes based in the nursery can be offered to children who have gone to school before the age of five.

The 'core and cluster' approach

This outreach approach has been developed by the Early Childhood Education Forum (1996) as a model for nursery expansion. The Forum visualises each community having at least one Centre, providing a range of services directly to children and families and supporting other non-centre provision in the community, through shared training, through being a reference point, and by providing a library and facilities that can be used by others. This approach extends the Centre's influence for the benefit of a larger population.

Appendix to Chapter 5

Terms and conditions of business

The following are the terms and conditions of business of ('the Company'). By signing the application form and applying for a place at one of the Company's nurseries ('the Nursery') you agree to be bound by these terms which can only be varied if such variation is agreed in writing and signed by an authorised representative of the Company.

1   Deposit
A deposit is payable and returnable to the Company with the application form. The deposit is held by the Company with the application until your child leaves the Nursery when (provided written notice of withdrawal has been given to the Company in accordance with paragraph 4 below and all fees and other charges are paid up to date) it will be refunded to you. Interest does not accrue on the deposit.

2   Acceptance
The Company will send a written acceptance of your application for a place at the Nursery. Deposits paid with applications that cannot be accepted will be refunded immediately.

3   Fees
3.1   Fees for each calendar month are payable in advance by direct debit on the 25th day of the previous calendar month.

3.2   Fees due for periods of part of a month at the beginning of your child's attendance at the Nursery are payable one month before your child's starting date and will be invoiced separately.

3.3   Fees due for periods of part of a month at the end of your child's attendance at the Nursery are payable by cheque on the 25th day of the month preceding your child's departure and will be invoiced separately.

3.4   Payment for extra hours for pre-school children and extra days for babies, toddlers and pre-school children which are needed on an ad hoc basis will be invoiced separately and are payable by cheque on or in advance of the date the extra hours or days are required.

3.5   Fees are payable throughout the period that your child is due to attend the Nursery and no rebate will be made for absence due to sickness, family holidays or any other reasons.

3.6   No refund of fees will be made if you postpone the date your child starts at the Nursery to a date later than the agreed starting date.

3.7   The Company reserves the right not to admit your child to the Nursery in the event of non-payment of fees or cancellation of your direct debit.

3.8   Fees are subject to review and can be increased at the Company's discretion without notice and at any time.

4   Notice of withdrawal/change in requirements
4.1   From the time the Company accepts your application for a place at the Nursery in accordance with paragraph 2 above three months written notice must be given to the Company (time to be of the essence) in order to:-
   4.1.1 withdraw your child from the Nursery;

4.1.2 delay or cancel your child's starting date at the Nursery;

4.1.3 decrease the number of hours in a day or days in a week that your child attends the Nursery.

4.2   Failure to give the required written notice in accordance with 4.1.1 and 4.1.2 above will result in fees being payable for the appropriate period in lieu of the full notice that should have been given.

4.3   Failure to give the required written notice in accordance with Clause 4.1.3 above will result in fees being payable for the original hours and/or days until the three months notice period would have expired if properly given.

4.4   Notice of withdrawal or change in requirements is deemed to commence on the date that the written notice is received by the Company.

4.5   If you wish to cancel your child's place at the Nursery following the Company's written acceptance in accordance with paragraph 2 but prior to your child starting at the Nursery and 3 months' notice is served by you to this effect in accordance with paragraph 4.1, the deposit paid with the acceptance form will be returned to you subject to an administration charge of £50.00.

5   Recovery of unpaid fees
The Company reserves the right to charge interest at the rate of 2% per cent per month on all outstanding fees. You will also be responsible for the payment of all additional charges incurred by the Company in the collection of outstanding fees including but not limited to our internal administrative charges and our solicitors' costs and disbursements.

6   Child's details
6.1   The Nursery requires and will rely on detailed information relating to your child as contained in the Company's consent and information form which shall form part of this contract. The Company must be immediately informed in writing of any changes to the information provided and is not liable for the consequences of your failure to update the information.

6.2   The Company will require you to fully complete and sign the consent and information form prior to leaving your child at the Nursery.

7   Removal of child
The Company reserves the right to require the removal of a child from the Nursery on a temporary or permanent basis at its discretion. In the event of permanent removal fees will be payable for the then current month but no further payments will be due in lieu of notice. No refund of fees will be made for temporary removal.

8   Generally
8.1   No failure or delay on behalf of the Company to exercise any right or remedy under these terms and conditions shall be construed or operate as a waiver.

8.2   This contract including all disputes hereunder shall be interpreted and resolved in accordance with the laws of England.

6

Working to a Plan

- Running a Nursery is Running a Small Business

- Business Planning

- Setting Objectives

- Understanding the Language of Finance

- Performance Measurement

- Sources of Finance

- Setting Fees

Running a Nursery is Running a Small Business

Whether you are the owner of your nursery or simply the manager, you should have an attitude towards the nursery as a small business in order to appreciate and be able to handle the conflicting pressures of quality and cost. The longstanding response of the private nursery sector to the criticism of being motivated by profit alone has been that providing a good service to the local community, raising standards for parents, and offering a service where none previously existed, is more likely to lead to profits being made than the provision of an inadequate service.

Coopers & Lybrand, the major accountancy firm, undertook a survey in 1991 which looked at the key motivators for anyone starting up and running a small business. The findings add credibility not only to the private nursery sector, but also to small businesses in general. When it comes to measuring success, 82% of small-business owners see the quality of their service as a very important factor, while 64% go for pure financial performance. The message is clear: quality and customer service are the keys to long-term prosperity. It is the combination of quality and financial performance that provides the best measure of success.

The Coopers & Lybrand study also seems to suggest that most owners of small companies have a healthy and personal desire to improve both the capital value and the financial performance of their firms, and don't just want to go for growth for growth's sake.

Once a business starts to grow the overheads can be spread over a wider base. Supplies and services can be bought in larger quantities and this usually means better terms and lower costs. The combination of these factors generally leads to a higher profit margin, which in turn provides funds to improve the way things are done in the business. This investment can lead to lower costs. This 'virtuous circle', as it is known, can make a growing business more cost competitive than one that is continuously marking time.

One of the pressing concerns in the nursery business is finding the money for training and service development, whilst holding fees down to a level that parents can afford. They can be budgeted for at the outset, with the corresponding uplift in fees, or they can be afforded once the nursery has accumulated surplus funds from its existing service. *Growing* the nursery, whether this means ensuring that it is full, or expanding, can offer some solution to the dilemma.

As well as having a cost advantage, a business can make other gains over its slower competitors. For example, launching a new service gives a nursery more to sell to its existing parent base. This strategy can make it more difficult for smaller competitors to break into that parent base, as they are perceived as having less to offer. This type of growth strategy can, if coupled with high-quality standards, lead to improved parent loyalty and a further push on the momentum of the virtuous circle.

Nursery managers may not be responsible for such strategic moves, but they need to be aware that these are the kinds of pressure the business will be responding to – and that means finding ways in which the nursery can incorporate the thinking.

Nursery managers will always be action-oriented, practical organisers. These are key requirements for the post. However, the application of these skills can be transformed if they can be related to the key objectives of the business, which may be the nursery itself, or it may be a broader organisation. This means understanding the *business plan*. A business plan may comprise a set of statements and columns of figures on one side of A4, or it may be a weighty reference document that is brought out of the drawer, dusted off, and reviewed by committee every few years. Whatever the format, the business plan places today's activities in the context of where the business is heading. If your nursery does not have one, it would be worthwhile to construct one. At the very least, it will help with responsibilities at management level. It will also help to ensure that activities have a purpose, and that one purpose is consistent with another.

Business Planning

The preparation of a business plan should not be a once-and-for-all exercise. The process of examining what you want to do and testing its viability is as important as the successful outcome and achievement of the plan itself.

As with any plan, a business plan enables you to drive your business forward, rather than being left to respond to the myriad of internal and external factors affecting everyday business life. It is this self-focus and analysis which lies at the heart of the process and is its most valuable and lasting aspect. However, a more usual imperative for the preparation of a business plan is the need to supply a bank with sufficient information on which to make a decision to lend you money. A third, and frequently overlooked, reason for preparing a business plan is to make clear to staff what is before the organisation – where it is aiming to be in the months and years ahead.

The most valuable use of my own business plan has been to provide me with a means of anticipating the effects of change. Reference points are important as a marker, against which new ideas can be measured. A business plan lays down such markers, and provides a basis on which to consider how changes will affect the business. In a way, a business plan is a series of layers of information. If a change requires you to adjust the top layer, it is probably something that can be incorporated into day-to-day activity quite easily. If, however, the change demands a reassessment at the deepest level, then the process of addressing the change may be painful, and touch on fundamental values.

A business plan should have three broad sections:

- A section on your service and the marketplace will cover what your service consists of and how it is distinctive. It will identify who your clients will be and why they need and are likely to buy the services you are to provide. The general marketing environment will be covered – is it a growth area, and who are your competitors? What will selling your service depend on – what are your critical success factors? This first section amounts to the *marketing plan.*
- The second part will focus on *how* the service will be delivered. An analysis of your own strengths and weaknesses will help to identify what other skills and experiences you will need to buy in and where you are likely to find them. Having decided on what your service consists of, you are in a position to calculate how many staff you will need to employ and the profile of the staff team. Assessing the capability of the whole staff team will lead to the need for computers, systems and procedures, and other *non-human* resources. You will then have your *resources plan.*
- Finally, you need to quantify what the marketing and resources plans imply in terms of funding, and what they will deliver in terms of revenue. The most critical aspect of this part of the business plan is to lay out your *planning assumptions –*

i.e. the basis on which you are going to collect and use income in the delivery of your service. How profitable will the operation be, and what will be the cash requirements of the organisation? And what if some of your planning assumptions are wrong? Just how wrong can you afford to be, and for how long, and what action can be taken to put it right?

Before going on to discuss a business plan in more detail, it is worth saying that the plan should be appropriate for the size of your business – it does not need to be a small volume! Its essential purpose is to demonstrate that you have thought through the issues of running your nursery as a business, that you have thought about the threats to stability it might face, and that the figures involved look sensible.

At this point many management books quote the experience of Anita Roddick, who was turned down flat by a bank on production of her first business plan, when asking for a £4000 loan to start up Bodyshop. The rest is part of business planning folklore!

Setting Objectives

At the beginning of every business planning cycle – i.e. when you set out and when you review the way in which you wish to move forward – you need to look at your prime objectives. If you cannot identify these, then that too tells you something.

Nursery nurses are used to planning. What is more, they are used to making plans on the basis of observation of the requirements of children. It is this same approach that the business plan needs. Why are you really doing this? What is your *mission* in running a nursery? This is the start of the planning process:

- A statement of mission
- A statement of objectives
- Identification of tasks
- Formulation of action plans

Note that mission statements and objectives are 'what' statements, whereas tasks and action plans are 'how to' statements – what to do on Monday morning.

Mission statements and objectives are *directional*, intended to focus your attention on the essentials that encapsulate your special *competencies* to deliver the service to the parents and children you intend to satisfy. It is through being very specific that a small business can differentiate itself from its larger competitors. This is often described as a *personal service* – a service that has not lost its distinctive character through becoming larger and sometimes less focused.

The mission statement

The mission statement should explain what business you are in and include some or all of the following:

- For *what* reason are you are doing this?
- *Who* are you trying to satisfy?
- With *what* services will you meet that demand?
- *How* will you deliver the services?
- *Where* will you be in the future?

Above all, mission statements should be realistic, achievable and brief. My own, prepared in 1992, is shown in Figure 22.

The mission statement of Ratners the jewellers, before the company went bankrupt, was:

'Ratners offer customers jewellery at prices they can afford rather than quality they cannot.'

Andrew Campbell, director of the London-based Ashbridge Strategic Management Centre, has said:

MISSION STATEMENT

- Our mission is to be the leading nursery provider in the UK, offering a premium service to working parents that is distinctive for its unique qualities and professional integrity.

- Our main purpose will be supported by the further developments of our innovative childcare strategy consultancy service in order that we remain at the forefront of the industry.

- Our business strategy is based on our commitment to people development. We see this as our most effective route to maintain our industry leader position.

Figure 22. A mission statement.

'Many of the world's outstanding companies employ people with what we call "a sense of mission". They believe that their company is special and they are proud to be a part of it.'

Campbell headed a research project into how managers can better understand and create a sense of mission in their organisations. He is convinced that firms increasingly need passionate employees, and says:

'Many organisations have become depersonalised to the point where energy levels are low, cynicism is high and work fails to excite or fulfil employees. We find that committed staff perform many times more effectively . . . '.

I think that, generally, such sentiments do not characterise a nursery team. In my experience, nursery staff feel passionately about what they do and have an exceptionally strong sense of commitment towards children and parents. But do they feel the same about nursery organisation? If the answer to this is No, then it is probably because the organisation has not shared its mission.

After a study of more than 100 statements from American, Japanese and European companies, the Ashbridge Centre concluded that these statements in themselves had little impact on business success. Much more important was whether a sense of mission already existed in the hearts and minds of employees. Employees not only need to have a clear understanding of what their company is trying to achieve, but also need to be emotionally committed to its aims before a meaningful statement can be written. If commitment is lacking, a mission statement is at best likely to be ignored and at worst treated with cynicism. From these findings, Campbell set out five principles to help managers trying to create a sense of mission (see Figure 23).

'Leaders should not forget that although a sense of mission is an emotional force it can be managed,' Campbell says. 'It is an aspect of business which cannot be ignored. An organisation with a sense of mission has a strong advantage.'

The objectives

Setting your objectives is about how you intend to fulfil your mission. It is your *success strategy* – how you will survive and thrive *and* remain true to your mission.

> 1. Leaders should pick a theme around which to develop a mission. It should capture the business' future strategy and values, and should be easy to translate into behaviour and standards.
> 2. Focus on action rather than words.
> 3. Standards and behaviour should clearly affirm the business' new direction.
> 4. Be patient – developing a mission takes years.
> 5. Build and sustain trust. This is often achieved by senior management being visible and open about changes taking place.

Figure 23.   Principles on which to create a sense of mission.

Most commonly, small businesses set their objectives in revenue terms: what do we want or need our income to be, and by when? However, for nurseries, the focus of attention is *occupancy* rather than *turnover*, as a measurement of business success.

You will need to set objectives under the following headings, and for the short term (18 months) and longer term:

- *Size*: How big do you want to be and by when?
- *Reputation*: What do you want people to think of your nursery?
- *Profitability*: What do you want to earn from it?
- *Future*: What are your longer term aspirations?

Your objectives may be very personal, particularly if you own the business (e.g. 'I want to ensure that in 5 years' time the nursery is profitable enough to be sold and to allow me to retire'). Or they may be less to do with you and more to do with growth of the business (e.g. 'I want to build our reputation for offering value for money services to working parents'), hence safeguarding your ability to take on workplace nursery contracts.

For your objectives to work they need to meet eight criteria:

- *They must be measurable.* You can get the business to where you want it to be only by setting specific targets. These need not always be financial, but may relate to a low staff turnover, or a percentage of the occupancy coming from the local residential community.
- *They should be realistic but challenging.* The objectives need to stretch everyone a little further than they want to go, but

within the boundaries of possibility. For example, if your goal is to pay nursery staff the best salaries, but your nursery fees are at the bottom of the league, it is unlikely that anyone will believe in your objectives.

- *They should have timescales.* Every objective should have a date set for its achievement. Becoming profitable 'as soon as possible' requires a very different approach from becoming profitable 'within 18 months'.
- *They require consultation.* People responsible for achieving objectives need to be involved in setting them, and they must understand that they are responsible for achieving them. As the nursery manager, you have the responsibility of indicating what you believe to be appropriate objectives, but you need to carry others with you.
- *They must be communicated.* Every team member needs to know where the nursery is headed and what they stand to gain if this is achieved. This is not necessarily money, but could be career development, broadened responsibility, or improved terms of employment.
- *They should be capable of monitoring against performance.* If not, people will think that you don't really care whether they are achieved or not.
- *They should be capable of being challenged.* Team members need to feel that they can challenge your objectives. You may like to invite them to prepare their own, and to compare achievability with yours.
- *They need to be updated.* Objectives are based on assumptions about the internal and external worlds of the nursery. The market you intended to serve may change: a local factory closes; a school suddenly opens its own nursery class; or revised registration requirements suggest a totally new staffing framework, involving you in additional costs.

Figure 24 gives a general indication of how small companies go about setting objectives. The results show that internal criteria are more of a driving force than market-led criteria.

Meeting your objectives

Although making detailed comparisons with the competition is

Comparison with key competitors	41%
Comparison with business sector overall	49%
Self-determined standards	66%
Company strategy	68%
Comparison with own previous performance	76%
Source: Peat Marwick (1990)	

Figure 24.   What are the objectives based on?

unlikely to be something you find terribly useful or central to what you do, you need to understand that parents will be doing just that.

We positively encourage parents to look around before making a final selection. This enables them to understand for themselves how our service differs and why our fees are what they are! Having looked at a number of others, if parents then make a positive choice in favour of our nursery, they are unlikely to waiver at a later date.

However, you can provide parents with information that helps them to see the differences between your nursery and others. Parents need to know how your service will benefit them and their child. They tend to be less interested in your perspective on child development or the academic underpinning for the nursery's philosophy. What we may feel proud of as elements of our service need to give way to the promises and guarantees we are prepared to offer parents.

Once you have established what you are offering, and to whom, you can make the *features* of your service be seen in terms of the *benefits* parents get when they book a place for their child. Features are what a service has or is; benefits are what the features mean for the parent and child.

The financial plan

The financial plan seeks to reflect the implications of your marketing and operational plans, in the form of profit-and-loss accounts, cash flows and balance sheets. Different strategies or variations of existing ones are tested to validate their effect on the project's financial performance.

Key assumptions	Basis of assumption	Confidence in assumption	What would happen if this assumption proved incorrect?
1			
2			
3			
4			
5			

Figure 25.   A table like this can be used to identify how robust your assumptions are.

The believability of any business plan will depend greatly on the assumptions that underpin it. These assumptions should cover the key areas of business and its operating environment. You also need to assess the downside risk and show how far things can go before new action has to be taken. Your assumptions can be recorded and monitored using a table like that in Figure 25.

Understanding the Language of Finance

Liquidators – who ought to know why businesses fail if anyone does – put 'lack of reliable financial information' at the top of their list. Many failed entrepreneurs believe accounting to be a bureaucratic nuisance carried out for the benefit of the Inland Revenue alone. These same people, who would never drive a car without a fuel gauge, speedometer, or oil pressure indicator, frequently set off at breakneck speed running their business only with a 'gut feeling' or perhaps the annual accounts to guide them. For them the end of the first year is often the end of the business.

Taking the analogy further, the motorist must also plan ahead to arrive successfully at the desired destination safely and on time. The success of any journey – particularly a long one – depends very much on the care taken at this stage. The preparation must centre around three distinct areas:

- the car: making sure it is serviced, filled with fuel, and generally in a fit state to make the journey;

- the route: choosing one that takes account of other traffic, possible roadworks, and facilities en route such as petrol, refreshments, etc.;
- the travellers: ensuring that everyone is prepared for the journey.

If this stage is accomplished with reasonable care and attention, the travellers and their vehicle have a very good chance of success in the next phase, which is the journey itself.

The most sound approach to the journey is to assess the distance to be travelled, determine an average travelling speed that is maintainable and safe, and from this determine the time needed to travel the distance. Then, working back from when you want to arrive, and allowing a margin of safety for petrol stops, refreshments, etc., you can calculate when you must set off. The rest of the journey should be plain sailing provided you follow your plan, follow the map correctly, and take account of the warning signs along the route. In all probability you will arrive at your destination safely and on time.

There are many parallels between planning a car journey and planning a business.

The balance sheet

You need a method of periodically measuring the growth and development of your venture. The balance sheet is a 'snapshot' which shows where the money came from to fund the business and where it was spent – at a fixed point in time, usually at annual intervals. The *where it came from* will usually include your own cash, share capital, the profit generated to date and loans received to date (both long-term and short-term). The *where it went to* will usually include fixed assets, stocks, debtors, plus the cash left in the *'tank'*. The comparison with motoring would be the milometer which measures the absolute distance the car has travelled, as opposed to the relative or changing performance measurement offered by the speedometer.

Profit-and-loss account

This is another moving picture of how well the business is doing, in terms of costs and profitability – usually prepared on a month-ly basis but covering an accounting period of one year. This can be compared to the speedometer in the car which constantly changes as the car progresses on its journey. The profit-and-loss account monitors the day-to-day performance of the business and gives the business person the information needed to identify the areas where corrective action should be taken – the equivalent of slowing down and taking notice of the road signs.

The business plan forecasts what these statements will look like at various points in the future. It is your first *operating budget*.

Operating budgets

A lot of businesses do not make a profit or have enough cash at the right time because the management has not planned ahead. Too often, they do not know how much profit or loss has been made until months after the end of the financial year. And often, profit is not properly thought out until there is a crisis.

Budgeting gives you a useful planning tool. By comparing your actual performance with the budget, you can spot difficulties early on and take action to put them right. However, all budgets are based on assumptions, so these must be specific and as realistic as possible.

In your operating budgets you can build-in contingencies to cover unexpected expenditure. A contingency can be shown as a separate item or included in the individual cost figures.

Costs

You must also be clear about the difference between the various costs of running your business. Some will vary depending on how well your business is doing. Some will not change.

Variable costs

Also known as 'direct costs', your variable costs are linked direct-ly to producing your service. They are the costs of your new ma-terials, and so on, as well as the wages of your employees who actually produce the service, i.e. not admin staff.

Fixed costs

You will have to meet these costs, even if you do not sell places. They include rent, rates, heating, lighting, insurance and fixed salaries, including your own. They are also known as 'indirect costs' or 'overheads'.

Depreciation

Depreciation takes into account the reduction in value of an asset over its working life. It is thus an expense, and so you should charge it to the profit-and-loss account, and include it in the operating budget.

Cash flow

This is a moving picture of how well the business is doing, in terms of cash movements. It bears a very close resemblance to the profit-and-loss account but reflects the effect the *credit taken from suppliers* and *given to customers* has on the cash in the business.

Profit does not always equal cash. Here the comparison with the car is particularly apt. A car needs petrol to run and the petrol gauge shows how much there is in the tank; a business needs cash to survive and the cash-flow statement shows how much there is in the business 'tank'.

Cash-flow forecasting

Once you have worked out an operating budget, you are ready to move on to produce a cash-flow forecast.

Unlike your operating budget, your cash-flow forecast is not to do with profit and loss. It is just your best estimate of how the cash will go in and out of your bank account over a certain period.

Cash is the lifeblood of your business. Managing cash badly is one of the main reasons for business failure. The time you spend working out your cash needs and monitoring cash flow is time well spent. This is because you can:

- find out when you might not have enough cash before it happens;
- find out when you might make extra cash and use it efficiently;
- make sure you have enough cash for any necessary capital expenditure;

- find out how to use your resources more efficiently and reduce costs.

Like your operating budget, your cash-flow forecast will be based upon assumptions. Again you must be realistic. Think about the best and worst cases and explain the assumptions you make. The more realistic your forecasts, the better any bank will like them.

- Think about the period of credit you will give to your customers or take from your suppliers. For example, suppose you can keep your customers to 30 days' credit (which will not be easy). Your *operating budget* could show the fees you invoiced, say, in January, but this cash should not be in your cash-flow projection until February – and then only if you are sure your customers will pay on time. If you have never had dealings with your suppliers before, you might have to settle their bills immediately. Obviously this will affect your cash flow – you will be buying things before your client pays for them.
- Your forecast should show all cash you will pay and receive, including your own salary, capital spending and loans. These are all part of your cash flow. However, depreciation is not, because it is only a notional book entry – it does not mean real cash coming in or going out of the business.
- VAT (value-added tax) will be shown in your cash-flow forecast but not in your operating budget. This is because it is not a charge against profit and loss, but a cash settlement.

Break-even analysis

With the information contained in the above financial statements, the manager will know whether the business has made a profit or loss in the past, but may not know whether it is still making a profit. A break-even analysis will show the level of sales required to generate sufficient profit to cover the overheads of the business, and thereby break even. The manager can then be confident that if he or she trades at above this break-even level of sales, the business will be operating profitably, barring any changes in the level of profit and overheads.

In car terms, the driver knows that in order to arrive at her destination on time she has to average so many miles per hour, say 50. If the driver averages less than 50 miles per hour, then she will be late; conversely if the driver exceeds it for any length of time she will arrive early. The 50 miles per hour is her break-even point. In business terms arriving early equals making a profit, and arriving late equals making a loss.

You need a clear appreciation from the outset that profit is not cash, and cash is not profit. In the short term, a small business can survive even if it is not making a profit, provided it has sufficient cash reserves, but it cannot survive for long without cash even though it may be making a profit. The purpose of the cash-flow projection is to calculate how much cash a business is likely to need to accomplish its objectives, and when it will need it. The projections will form the basis of negotiations with any potential provider of capital.

An example

The example below looks at the simplified finances of Caroline Graham. She has become a little confused by the complexity of her financial affairs, and has decided to get things sorted out. In short, she wants to know where she stands.

The list below tells us something of Caroline's circumstances, but until we reorganise the information we cannot really understand her true financial position:

Cash	£50
House	£50 000
Mortgage	£45 000
Money owed by sister (Jackie)	£135
Overdraft	£100
Car	£1 000
Credit card	£50
Jewellery and paintings	£350
Hire purchase (on various goods)	£500
Furniture	£500

Caroline believes that, in money matters, things divide neatly into two types: amounts that you have and amounts that you owe, with the latter usually exceeding the former. Using this concept we can show the same information in the following manner. The

Liabilities and claims (where she got the money from)		Assets (what she has done with the money)	
	£		£
Overdraft	100	Cash	50
Mortgage	45 000	House	50 000
Hire purchases	500	Car	1 000
Credit card	50	Jewellery and paintings	350
Total claims by other people	45 650	Money owed by sister	135
		Furniture	500
C's capital	6 385		
Total of C's and other people's capital	52 035	C's assets	52 035

Figure 26.   Caroline Graham's finances.

right-hand side of Figure 26 shows Caroline's assets – what she has done with the money she has had. The left lists where she got the money from to pay for these assets – the liabilities and claims against her.

She has acquired £52 035's worth of assets and must have provided an identical sum from one source or another. As we can find only £45 650 owed to other people, the only reasonable assumption is that Caroline herself must have put her past income towards buying the assets.

Now, while Caroline might be happy with the help we have given her so far, it is unlikely she will be completely satisfied. Like the rest of us, she probably considers events as long term or short term in nature. Even though we have shown a fairly dazzling picture of £52 035 of assets, she knows she is short of cash for day-to-day living. So, once again, we can restructure the information on her financial position to give a clearer picture.

In Figure 27 we can now see that her short-term financial position is dominated by the money owed by the sister. If that is safe, then all current liabilities can be met. If it is not safe and the money is unlikely to be repaid quickly, the position is not so good. There is an accounting convention according to which 'current liabilities' are those that we will have to pay within a year. Similarly 'current assets' will turn into cash within a year.

Liabilities and claims (where she got the money from)		Assets (what she has done with the money)	
	£		£
Mortgage	45 000	House	50 000
Hire purchase	500	Car	1 000
C's capital	6 385	Jewellery and paintings	350
	———	Furniture	500
	51 885		———
			51 850
Current liabilities (short-term)		Current assets (short-term)	
Overdraft	100	Money owed by sister	135
Credit cards	50	Cash	50
	———		———
	150		185
	———		———
Total liabilities	**52 035**	**Total assets**	**52 035**

Figure 27.   Caroline Graham's 'balance sheet' today.

Figure 27 is very close to a balance sheet of Caroline's financial position.

Performance Measurement

The most important reason for having plans becomes clear when you begin to evaluate performance against them. To know that you are on track, where you and others expect you to be, is tantamount to your success as a manager. A recognised way of assessing financial performance is by the use of *key ratios*.

A ratio is something expressed as a proportion of something else. For example, a percentage is a ratio, where something is compared with a base of 100.

Key ratios point to questions about the business that need answers. They allow a manager to choose, from the hundreds of questions that might be asked, the handful that are really worth answering. In a small business, time is at a premium. This quick pre-selection is essential.

What are the key ratios?

Bear in mind that *profitability* is sales income or value of services sold, *minus* the cost of sales (i.e. everything that has gone into delivering that service – these are the direct or variable costs), i.e. the costs that are incurred entirely because of the service being supplied. For example, rent would be incurred whatever the business was supplying; staff in ratio to children would be employed only for a nursery service.

Gross profit ratio

Deduct the cost of sales from sales, and express the result as a proportion of sales by dividing by sales.

Operating profit ratio

Deduct overheads from the gross profit, and divide by sales. Overheads are your indirect or fixed costs.

This ratio demonstrates the importance of profit, whereas increased sales are not meaningful in themselves. If the ratio is too low, the manager should perhaps be looking for savings in administration, or ensuring that marketing effort is more closely targeted to result in higher occupancy.

Liquidity ratio

This ratio checks your cash position, whether you have enough working capital and whether you can meet your debts as they fall due.

'Debtors + cash' divided by 'creditors' should be 1:1. A lower ratio is risky. A higher ratio indicates that too much money is owed to you or that your borrowing is too high. Either way you are taking an unnecessary level of financial risk, and suppliers may stop supplying or even petition for bankruptcy.

Because the cash position is critical in a small business, creditor and debtor policies are very important.

How many times can you cover current liabilities? 'Debtors + cash' divided by 'bills and interest due' should be 1:1. A lower ratio is risky. A much higher ratio indicates that too much money is owed to you or that your borrowing is too high.

Sources of Finance

Two sources of funds are most commonly used:

- lenders;
- investors, including yourself.

Anyone lending money to, or investing in, a venture will expect the entrepreneur to have given some thought to the lender's or investor's needs, and to have explained how they can be accommodated in the business plan.

Banks, and indeed any other sources of debt capital, look for asset security to back their loans, and the near certainty of getting their money back. They charge an interest rate that reflects current market conditions and their view of the risk level of the proposal. Depending on the nature of the business in question and the purpose for which the money is being used, banks will take a five- to fifteen-year view.

As with a house mortgage repayment, banks will usually expect a business to start repaying both the loan and the interest on a monthly or quarterly basis immediately the loan has been granted. In some cases a capital 'holiday' for up to two years can be negotiated, but in the early stage of any loan the interest charge makes up the lion's share of repayments.

The lending bank will hope that the business will be a success so that it can lend more money in the future and provide more banking services such as insurance, tax advice, etc. to a loyal customer. The bank will be less interested in rapid growth and the consequent capital gain than in a steady stream of earnings almost from the outset.

As most new or fast-growing businesses generally do not make immediate profits, money for such enterprises must come from elsewhere. Risk or equity capital, as other types of funds are called, comes from venture capital houses (as well as being put in by founders, their families and friends). Because the inherent risks involved in investing in new and young ventures are greater than for investing in established companies, venture capital fund managers have to offer their investors the chance of larger overall returns. To do that, fund managers must not only keep failures to a minimum, they have to pick some big winners too – ventures with annual compound growth rates above 50% – to offset the inevitable mediocre performers.

Typically, from any ten investments a fund manager would expect one star, seven also-rans, and two flops. However, it is important to remember that, despite this outcome, venture capital fund managers are looking only for winners, so unless you are projecting high capital growth, the chances of getting venture capital are against you.

Not only do venture capitalists look for winners, they also look for a substantial shareholding in your business. There are no simple rules for what constitutes a fair split, but *Venture Capital Report*, a UK monthly publication of investment opportunities, suggests the following starting point:

For the idea	33%
For the management	33%
For the money	34%

It all comes down to how badly you need the money, how risky the venture is, how much money could be made – and your skills as a negotiator. However, it is salutary to remember that 100% of nothing is still nothing, so all parties to the deal have to be satisfied if it is to succeed.

A venture capital firm may also want to put a non-executive director on the board of your company to look after its interests. You will then have at your disposal a talented financial brain, so be prepared to make use of him or her. This service will not be free – you will either pay 'up front' in the fee for raising the capital, or you will pay an annual management charge.

As a fast-growing company typically has no cash available to pay dividends, investors can profit only by selling their shareholdings. With this in mind the venture capitalist needs to have an exit route in view at the outset, such as the Stock Exchange or a potential corporate buyer. Unlike many entrepreneurs (and some lending banks) who see their ventures as life-long commitments to success and growth, venture capitalists have a relatively short time horizon. Typically they aim to liquidate small company investments within three to seven years, allowing them to pay out individual investors and to have funds available for tomorrow's winners.

So, to be successful your business finances must take account of the needs of these two types of sources of finance. The factors are summarised in Figure 28.

Lenders (any safe bet)	Investors (winners only)

• Security and low risk
• 5–15-year horizon
• Ability to pay back loan and interest immediately
• conservative growth
• Small sums, with frequent top-ups
• No share of future profits, but want a loyal long-term customer
• No management involvement
	• High risk but high returns
	• 3–7-year horizon
	• 35% compound growth minimum, but no payments until the end of the deal
	• Large sums, with few top-ups
	• Substantial shareholding:
	  – for the idea 33%
	  – for management 33%
	  – for money 34%
	• Exit route evident at outset:
	  – back to founders
	  – trade buyer
	  – USM etc.
	• Hands-on involvement

Figure 28.   Factors to bear in mind with lenders and investors.

Getting a grant

Another source of money is neither debt nor equity, and in theory is free. The magic money source is called a 'grant'. The EU, the UK government and many local authorities give grants for one purpose or another. Various estimates put the total figure of grant aid available at between £500 million and £2 billion a year. *Sources of Grant Aid for Business in the UK* is a 2000-page, looseleaf and regularly updated guide to grants, published by Weka Publishing Ltd, 74–80 Camden Street, London NW1 1YW.

Before you rush off and search for this 'free money', do remember that someone giving a grant often wants you to do something that does not make commercial sense. There may be millions of pounds available to encourage you to set up your satellite production facility in an area that is currently populated by sheep; the grant may or may not compensate you for being miles from markets and potential employees.

The golden rule is: Decide what you want to do and check that it makes sound business sense; then see if anyone will fund you to do it.

Setting Fees

When considering what fee levels should be, the most frequent mistake is to set them too low. This can occur either through failing to understand all the costs associated with planning and delivering the service, or through yielding to the temptation to undercut or certainly not exceed fees charged by other nurseries. Both are usually fatal.

The nursery manager is the very best source of information on fees. The manager sees parents, hears their response to fees as quoted, and hears them compare the fees with those of other nurseries visited and other forms of childcare. It is useful to devise a form for feedback for those parents who visit but do not take up a place at the nursery, as it is equally very easy to blame price, when actually the reasons may be more complex.

There are internal and external issues that need to be considered when setting fees.

Internal issues

Costs

Make sure you have identified *all* the costs you are likely to incur in planning and delivering your service. Surprisingly this is often forgotten. If staff are going to have non-contact time for observation and activity planning, cover will need to be supplied if the nursery is to remain open. If there are to be 'inset' training days, then there is a cost to be covered, although fees may not be chargeable because the nursery will be closed.

Quality of service

The positioning of the service in the market is influenced largely by the fees/quality relationship. This is shown in Figure 29.

A confident approach would be to position the nursery in (4), (7) or (8) because they offer high value for money. Strategies (2), (3) and (6) may suit the short term but are unlikely to be sustainable over time.

Policy

The overall image you want to portray will also influence the fees you wish to charge.

	Low fees	Medium fees	High fees
Low quality	Cheap value (1)	Out of step (2)	Exploitive (3)
Medium quality	Above-average value (4)	Middle of road (5)	Overcharging (6)
High quality	Superb value (7)	High value (8)	Premium (9)

Figure 29.   The fees/quality relationship.

Running a nursery is not typical in business terms. Registration under the Children Act requires a certain level of costs to be incurred and a certain quality of service to be delivered. There are no serious and sustainable, cheap and cheerful nursery businesses. If parents regard the Children Act levels as par, then anything over and above the cheapest service they have come across needs to justify its higher prices. It is also a business in which 'gloss' in any form is seen to detract from the real benefits to children.

Where nurseries maintain fees at levels that barely cover costs, a number of people have undoubtedly been discouraged from starting new nurseries. In areas where nurseries have charged higher fees, new competitors have been attracted into the market.

Capacity

Capacity to provide childcare places will also influence fees charged. How fast the nursery will fill is a key factor in whether the nursery is viable and should not be underestimated in its importance. It is also important to remember that, once full, no more places can be sold. This is another factor that distinguishes the nursery business from many other small-business operations. Fees must be set at a level that will work, or can be reached, when the nursery is full, as well as when it is starting out. What will your fees need to be to cover your (high proportion of) fixed costs at the outset? Will this be higher than it needs to be when you are at 50%/85% full, and how will you handle that? Will you operate at a loss to begin with, or will you plan to make a proportionately higher return as the nursery fills?

External issues

Parents' perceptions

Because childcare has grown up in this country through the strong traditions of the public and voluntary sectors, it is only relatively recently that the true costs of providing nursery services have become general knowledge. Parents' opinion of value may still bear little or no relation to the cost, and because there are still many areas of the country that have little or no provision they may have little knowledge of competitive charges.

Fees convey a message to parents – that the service is 'budget', 'middle of the road' or 'top drawer'. Parents use fees to confirm their impression of the service and thereby make a choice. In this way, when you set a fee, you select the market of parents you wish to target. The three terms used above are difficult to use in relation to nursery services. 'Top drawer', as indicated by fees charged, in the view of many commentators would simply imply a service to which all children are entitled and which discerning parents should expect.

Competition

It is usually a misconception to think that new nurseries can undercut fees charged by established competitors. This is probably based on a misunderstanding of the real overheads and a lack of appreciation that 'unit' costs fall in proportion to experience – i.e. the time needed to undertake a task when you are experienced at it and have developed a system, in contrast to the first attempts.

Clearly it is important to take account of what competitors charge, because this provides an indication of what parents expect to pay. But fees are the easiest element of business to vary. The competition could follow you down the fees curve, forcing you into failure, far more easily than you could capture their parents with lower fees.

Business conditions

The overall conditions in the marketplace will have a bearing on setting fees, although it is not an industry in which parents 'shop around' for keener prices alone. In times of recession parents will (and did) question fees more than at other times; but because so high a proportion of costs – and therefore fees – is devoted to staff costs, parents can usually discern from the impression they get from staff, and the service they observe, whether the fee matches the service. If there are more staff around, and the nursery appears calm and uncluttered, and the children are engaged in activities, most parents will appreciate that there will be a correspondingly high fee level, in comparison with a nursery that does not have this appearance.

Parents are rightly wary of 'cut price' childcare, because the fees must also imply that Children Act standards are being cut, and therefore that the nursery is operating outside the legal requirements set down.

For me, the most important issue around fees is that they should not be blamed by nursery staff for lapses in performance. Given that fees for childcare are high – for every parent – it is very simple to say that bookings are not being made because prices are too high. Some parents will not be able to afford the fees and are unlikely to visit if this is their position. However, if after being appraised of the fees the parents visit the nursery, they are then confirming that the service in some way justifies the fees.

A second important issue is not to be over-anxious to correct an imbalance in budgets through increasing fees. As has already been noted, childcare costs are extremely high in any event, and all parents find them hard to afford. Increasing them even further is inevitably to run the risk of losing some children. Compare the effects of:

- a 5% increase in fees;
- a 5% cut in overheads;
- a 5% increase in booked places.

Increasing fees may not always be the appropriate response, and in my experience the other two are *always* worth attempting first. More subtle ways of using pricing would be to vary fees for different services or slots in the week, and to offer prepayment or 'off season' discounts during the summer holiday.

Finally, here is a setting-fees checklist:

- Set fee objectives.
- Don't set fees arbitrarily or by 'feel'.

- Relate fees to your marketing objectives, e.g. when you want to break even, how competitive you want to be, the image you wish to portray.
- Understand market conditions.
- Understand sensitivity to fees by parents.
- Outwit your competitors.

7

Reviewing the Service

- Responding to Parents

- Managing Change

- Quality Assurance

- Employing Consultants

- Using Advisers

Responding to Parents

According to the Confederation of British Industry, those who pay for pre-school care and education spend an average of 25% of earnings on the services they procure. If this is what parents are committing themselves to, they want and will see that their hard-earned money is well spent. What do parents expect and wish to see?

Rather than thinking or hoping that the priorities of parents are the same as those of providers, we should look at what they actually are. Susan Hay Associates Ltd undertook just such a survey amongst parents within the five nurseries that the company runs in the London area. It is important to note that the company's provision is 'Nurseries', and not 'Nursery Schools' or 'Pre-Preps'.

This distinction is drawn to emphasise the diversity within provision currently made in the independent sector. Indeed the sector's strength lies in the diversity and range of services offered to parents and children. The different labels suggest choice, but do they offer a basis on which services can be compared by parents? How do parents perceive the differences between the various labels placed on the service, and how do their expectations of the service differ because of the label used?

The objectives of the survey were to look at:

- how parents' priorities change as a baby grows and develops into a pre-school child;
- what outcomes are expected from a child's time at nursery.

The sample included the responses of approximately 120 sets of parents/carers, using one of five nurseries either in inner or outer London. The nurseries are largely used by working parents/carers, about half of whom receive large fee subsidies from their employers. The nurseries are located in both residential and workplace settings, and draw on a broad catchment of people working on site, locally, and commuting in to the West End or City.

Parents were asked to rate the importance of different aspects of the service for babies, toddlers and children about to transfer to school, under a number of developmental headings. The tables below list the given aspects of service together with the primary findings. Even though they each serve very different constituencies in terms of employer support and demographic profile, the three aspects of service given top priority in every section were the same from each parent group.

> **FOR YOUR CHILD AT EACH STAGE – BABY, TODDLER AND PRE-SCHOOL – WHICH OF THE FOLLOWING FEATURES DO YOU FEEL ARE MOST IMPORTANT IN THE NURSERY SERVICE?**

Given aspects of service:

Free choice of activities
Parent participation
Identifiable underlying educational principles
Continuity of staff
Effective senior management
Care routines
Integrated activities
Broad choice of activities
Health and safety procedures
Continuous programme of training for staff
Mixed age groupings
Adaptability to individual needs of child
Space and equipment
Qualifications of staff
Range of experience in staff team

Findings:

Babies	1	*Continuity of staff*
	2	*Health and safety procedures*
	3	*Care routines*
Toddlers	1	*Space and equipment*
	2	*Continuity of staff*
	3	*Effective senior management*
Pre-school	1	*Adaptability to individual needs of child*
	2	*Identifiable underlying educational principles*
	3	*Broad choice of activities*

WHAT ARE THE MOST IMPORTANT ASPECTS OF SERVICE FOR YOUR CHILD'S INTELLECTUAL DEVELOPMENT?

Given aspects of service:

Constant adult/child interaction
Teaching qualifications of staff
Early numeracy programme
Wide range of activities
Mixed age groups
Early science programme
Individual attention
Early literacy programme
Monitoring and observations

Findings:

Babies	*1*	*Constant adult/child interaction*
	2	*Individual attention*
	3	*Wide range of activities*
Toddlers	*1*	*Wide range of activities*
	2	*Constant adult/child interaction*
	3	*Mixed age groups*
Pre-school	*1*	*Wide range of activities*
	2	*Constant adult/child interaction*
	3	*Early literacy programme*

WHAT ARE THE MOST IMPORTANT ASPECTS OF SERVICE FOR YOUR CHILD'S SOCIAL AND EMOTIONAL DEVELOPMENT?

Given aspects of service:

Key-person system
Discipline policy
Mixed age groups
Equal opportunities policy

Individual attention
Care routines, esp. mealtimes
Parental participation
Range of experience in staff team
Children's work displays
Spatial environment
Outings and links with wider community

Findings:

Babies	1	*Individual attention*
	2	*Care routines, esp. mealtimes*
	3	*Key-person system*
Toddlers	1	*Mixed age groupings*
	2	*Key-person system*
	3	*Individual attention*
Pre-school	1	*Outings and links with wider community*
	2	*Discipline policy*
	3	*Key-person system*

> **WHAT OUTCOMES OF YOUR CHILD'S TIME AT NURSERY DO YOU FEEL ARE OF GREATEST BENEFIT AS THEY TRANSFER TO SCHOOL?**

Given aspects of service:

Letter recognition
Long concentration span
Participative play with other children
Taking and waiting turns
Knowing alphabet
Happy memories of nursery
Ability to count to 20
Participative play with adults
Musical awareness
Ability to speak confidently in front of others
Eager anticipation of school
Washing, dressing, toileting on own

Caring for younger children
Movement and dance awareness
Courtesy and manners

Findings:

1   *Participative play with other children*
2   *Speaking confidently in front of others*
3   *Happy memories*
4   *Eager anticipation of school*
5   *Courtesy and manners*
6   *Extended concentration span*

* * *

Few people question that parents must be encouraged to participate in the care and early learning of their child when it is entrusted to others. It follows that parents must be increasingly aware of the service offered, and that the service must appeal to the priorities of parents. The findings of the survey have helped us to look afresh at what we offer in our nurseries, and to understand better the special and separate role of the nursery, as well as its position as a stepping stone for the child. They have helped us to focus, not on what we as professionals believe is the best way forward, but rather to view our service from the parents' point of view and to integrate this into our planning process. Our review has concentrated on the following issues:

• Constant adult/child interaction and conversation, and the impact of a key-person system for children, are continuous requirements throughout nursery life.
• The benefits of what we offer are to provide the children with the ability to participate with others in constructive play, and to be confident in their choices and activities.
• If we are to present ourselves as offering a real option at pre-school age (i.e. ages 3–5), we must be able to demonstrate the principles that underpin our educational approach as well as our managerial ability to put these principles into practice effectively and efficiently.
• We must be able to offer the assurance to parents that our curriculum is built around their priorities and that there is evidence of these being addressed on a continuous basis. We must

be able to measure the effectiveness of attending to the identified priorities in terms of the children's development, and in a language that parents can share.

In addressing the issues raised by the survey we must acknowledge that there is a huge range of skills involved in taking them forward: teaching, caring, managing, organising, reviewing, and communicating.

Armed with these skills we need to rise to the challenge of continually reviewing parents' needs and desires for the care and education of their young children, and particularly at critical times within the period when the service is required – e.g. for the first baby of the family; when a second child is born; as babyhood is left behind; and when a child is approaching the time when they will transfer to school.

We also need to consider the match between what the nursery offers at these times and the actual needs, desires and priorities of parents. Finally, we need to examine parents' perceptions of the ways in which the service should develop, and how they can be addressed.

The survey enabled us to get a glimpse of the key discriminators in the decision-making process of parents faced with purchasing early years' services. It has told us something of how and when parents draw and redraw the boundaries in terms of what the service should offer. It did not address the fundamental issue of cost.

Managing Change

Change has become recognised as a necessary component of modern management. It has even become fashionable and in danger of becoming an end in itself.

Development is change and learning in balance. It is a fundamental law of ecology that, for any living thing to survive, its rate of learning must be equal to or greater than the rate of change in its environment. The external environment in which nurseries operate is changing rapidly – politically, socially, economically and academically. We should not increase the turbulence this will cause by over-emphasising the change side of the equation, at the expense of *learning*.

Change, is, after all, part and parcel of a nursery service. If we accept that our service must be parent-based, flexible to individual children's needs, creative and responsive, people-oriented, effective and efficient, it follows that every day is different, every moment incorporates changes.

So why do we need to address or cope with change as a discrete area of concern? This is because, sometimes:

- things do not turn out as expected;
- a policy or practice is not working properly;
- a new directive is imposed;
- a new development is discovered;
- change is worthwhile for change's sake.

In other words, changes occur for different reasons. Sometimes change is thrust upon us and at other times we introduce it ourselves. Some of the reasons may be negative. For example, changes made to budgets may be in order to redress a disappointing trend in the accounts; modifications in the activity programme may reflect the impossibility of having sufficient staff to cover all areas of the nursery at one time.

A new ruling may be introduced by the local authority that adds to their registration requirements, and restricts the service to children in a way you would prefer not to have to take on board.

On the positive side, new research into the way children develop may bring about a review of your curriculum, your child observation practice, or the qualities you look for in new staff. A new shift-pattern formula may result in more time for staff discussion with parents. A new member of staff with expertise in a specialist area, say equal opportunities, may introduce radical new approaches to positive image development.

What is our response to change? Usually it puts us into a state of shock, to one extent or another ('Why is this change necessary at all?'). Secondly, we are likely to make a defensive retreat ('Was this really necessary? What is wrong with the way we have been doing it up until now?'). Gradually we begin to acknowledge that the change is probably appropriate, and finally we adapt to it. This process can be handled in order to achieve a change quickly, or slowly, and it can be managed well, or badly.

Generally, people are willing to accept change if they have confidence in themselves in their role, and in their immediate seniors and colleagues, and in the management.

As a manager, you will have a management style, a way of

approaching and handling people and tasks, to achieve your objectives. The way changes are introduced into your setting will largely reflect your management style, and you will be judged as being effective or ineffective by others in terms of the introduction of change, in relation to your style. Figure 30 provides a scale on which you can assess the way you are inclined towards a particular approach.

The nature of change

Being action-oriented, managers of early years' services want to know 'how can I do this now?'. We have noted earlier the

BASIC STYLE	EFFECTIVE	INEFFECTIVE
HIGH TASK	Seen as knowing what he/she wants and imposing her/his methods for accomplishing this without creating resentment	Seen as having no confidence in others; unpleasant, and interested only in short-run output
HIGH TASK AND RELATIONSHIP	Seen as good motivator who sets high standards; treats everyone differently (as equals) and prefers team management	Seen as a person who tries to please everyone and so vacillates back and forth to avoid pressures from either side
HIGH RELATIONSHIP	Seen as having implicit trust in people; primarily concerned with developing the talents of her/his staff	Seen as primarily interested in harmony and being a 'good person'; unwilling to risk disruption of a relationship to accomplish a task
LOW TASK AND LOW RELATIONSHIP	Seen as appropriately permitting her/his subordinates to decide how the work should be done; and playing only a minor part in their social interaction	Seen as uninvolved and passive, as a 'paper shuffler', who cares little about the task at hand or the people involved

Figure 30.   Basic leader behaviour styles.

disastrous effects that introducing change too quickly can bring. Change is a process of nurturing and bringing out, rather than one of rushing on and hammering in.

Pedler *et al.* (1989) defined the 'learning organisation' (or the organisation best equipped to cope with change) as 'an organisation which *facilitates* the learning of all its members and *continuously* transforms itself'. There are links with training here, but there are dangers:

> 'Training is a liability in situations where you have to flex quickly – what price the training you had yesterday because today I want you to do something different? But you will not do it because you are so wedded to what we trained you to do yesterday!' – Nick Georgiades, British Airways

Change involves having a respect for all new ideas and valuing what each individual can bring, if given the opening:

> 'The first thought is that it is [change] about a company, as a priority objective, developing all its human resources, enhancing all their skills . . . but not being content with that . . . learning from those people how the company can be improved . . . so that it becomes a cycle of learning.' – Paul Marsh, Jaguar

The rate of external change on early years' services is increasing rapidly. With competition and deregulation being encouraged by the government, childcare providers are continually having to transform themselves to offer higher quality, more affordable and relevant services. Not all of them will make it. Those that do will have realised that the people with the ability to learn what their parents want, and who can respond rapidly to deliver it, will be those who contribute to add value and profitability to the services of the organisation, and ultimately, through the parents' increased perception of the quality of the services, their share of the market.

If people are unready or unprepared for change they will consider it as a problem, and their response will swing between absolute rejection and poor performance in what they are doing. The appropriateness and sensitivity with which change is introduced is frequently of larger concern than the change itself. A well-developed process is the 9-point plan.

1. Getting an authentic picture of the present

This requires us to distance ourselves from the present (problem) to which we have contributed in part, in order that we can openly face the necessary change. We need to create a risk-free environment in which to discuss the issue; that is, not one of criticism or reproach, but 'We are where we are, and where do we go from here?', as my chairman, Harry Salmon, likes to put it.

2. Developing a common vision

If the majority will commit to a common vision of the future in which they have had a hand, then there is a good chance of creating sufficient organisational energy to achieve it.

The purpose of the change needs to be shared, and it needs to be seen as contributing to, not compromising, the overall objective. Until all staff can share in the overall objective, they may well feel that their particular role is compromised by the change they are being asked to absorb ('We can no longer do what we set out to do in the intended way'). However, what they may not have understood is that, when the change was accepted, they would not have been able to do it at all!

3. Building a bridge between the present and the future

The best way to introduce a change is to draw on a coalition of:

- who *knows* about the problem (the cause);
- who *cares* about the problem (the effect);
- who *can do* anything about the problem (the solution).

4. Launching a 'pilot'

Another way of introducing a change is to test the change within a small group or over a short period of time. This will provide an opportunity for staff to shape the change themselves from the very practical standpoint of 'Does this work better than it did before?'. It will also provide an opportunity to get it right from the outset, rather than risk the upheaval of change, only to find that a further modification is required to see it successfully in place.

5. Communicating the change

There is rarely any benefit in keeping things secret, but there are often disbenefits. For instance, others are denied the opportunity to introduce a good idea, they are precluded from the energy generated from something that works well, they are not given the chance to enthuse.

If the process is shared, then so too is the rigour with which the change is being considered. It has not come about on a whim, or even a prayer, but a well thought-out developed improvement.

6. Encouraging others to join

People have different reasons for involving themselves in the process of change. Some will want to ensure that the balance of micro-politics is not jolted, that territory is not given up to others. Most want to contribute to the greater good of the nursery and enjoy being involved in finding the right solution.

One Japanese company reports that it implements over 5000 staff suggestions per day. How many has your organisation implemented this year?

7. Reinforcing corporate culture

Charles Handy (1987) would say that the culture in your organisation is likely to be broadly based on one of the following:

- *one-manager rule*, where information is kept centrally, and the centre cannot easily be challenged;
- *the role culture*, where everyone knows their place and all responsibilities are standardised and accepted, and is slow to change;
- *the task culture*, where people take on specific projects, with deadlines and agreed objectives, releasing a lot of energy from a few individuals;
- *the people culture*, where the focus is on each person being treated equally, but no one individual being able to take a lead.

It is unlikely that your nursery is purely one or another. However, the way change is received will largely be determined by which culture is dominant.

Some key questions to staff could help you identify the broader perception of the nursery:

- What objectives would they use to describe the organisation?
- How would they describe what they would like it to be in the future?

- What happens when things go wrong?
- Who gets rewards and why?
- What releases most energy within the team?

8. Rewarding achievers and others

Commitment from staff is discussed in more detail in Chapter 4, and the relative perceived reward method. Everyone seeks recognition to show that they are a valued part of the organisation. It is the manager's role to ensure that this is positive recognition and in line with the organisation's objectives. 'What can I do to make your work more effective?' can illicit important information for the manager in terms of supporting staff in their response to change.

9. Feedback on the manager's behaviour

Staff are likely to respond best to a manager whose words and action are synchronised. This sounds easy, but many managers expect people to do what they are told, often with little reference to other decisions. It is then not surprising that responses are sometimes contradictory. The recent 'scandal' of large pay rises for directors of the formerly nationalised industries, alongside cost-cutting and redundancies across the board, are a case in point.

Conditions for change

We have already looked at what might constitute an external or an internal change. But there is another type of discussion that affects both the way changes may be introduced and the response such changes will attract.

Early years' services are re-framing themselves almost daily, as this is written. The proposed government childcare voucher scheme, due to take effect in April 1997 and currently in its pilot phase, has given rise to a total overhaul of the inspection system, new definitions of education in under-fives settings, renewed interest in quality assurance schemes, and a heightened awareness amongst parents of both their children's entitlement and their own expectations of providers.

It is a time of radical policy change, as providers have little chance of directly influencing such disruption. Instead, they must consider how to respond within the context of their organisation;

they must *learn* how to adapt what they do to the needs of the current environment. In Bob Garratt's (1990) terms, this is part of the policy cycle of organisational learning. Here the manager is rising above day-to-day routines, giving thoughtful leadership and direction as current information is sifted, and in the face of *coups* such as the recent government intervention.

At the operations level, people tend to be so busy and 'heads down' in the nursery that their responses to problems tend to be to do more of or less of what is already happening. This is particularly true when targets or budgets are tightened and priorities have to be readjusted. Performance is monitored against plans and appropriate action is taken through the control systems (see Figure 31 and Chapter 6). Ideally, the whole is run like a well-oiled machine – were it not for the deviations from plans that break into the rhythm with unfailing regularity! It is managing these deviations back on to plans that provides the manager with his or her most essential task.

Effects of change

One of the direct consequences of belonging to an industry providing a service in which there are so many stakeholders is that the effect of any change must also be measured in terms of each of their interests. Most directly affected will be children, parents and staff. However, commercial life requires that shareholders, employers and developers may also have their situation changed by what is being introduced.

The reason for the change may be compelling for some shareholders, but may be unmeasurable for others. This strengthens the case for consultation on the change.

Shareholders are in the best position to alter the effect on themselves of a change. However, you must be certain about what you are consulting on, in order that their involvement has credibility. Have you decided already, or are you *consulting* on:

- the notion of the change;
- the options for change;
- the mechanics of the preferred option?

Either of these may be appropriate, but there are few more frustrating situations to be in than being asked your opinion, only to find that the decision has already been taken and that your approval is all that is being sought.

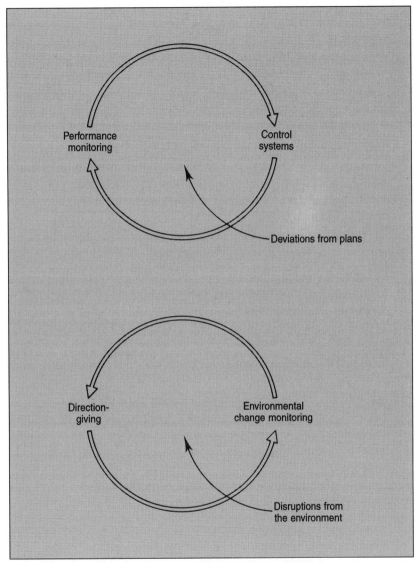

Figure 31.   Organisational learning: the operational and policy cycles.

In some instances it may be inappropriate to consult at all. This may be where one stakeholder will inevitably have to stomach a difficult change, for the sake of other stakeholders. It may also arise where individuals find it compromising to be party to a change, and would prefer to abstain (silently).

Quality Assurance

Being a professional carries privileges but also liabilities. In recent years, as the law has favoured the consumer over the provider of services where a doubt exists, and when deregulation has taken precedence over tighter controls, professionals of all kinds have needed to demonstrate that they can be self-regulating; that discernible steps are taken to evidence their competence in practice. The fundamental rule is that, having told a parent what your service consists of, you must match their expectations with what is actually provided. Being able to demonstrate that what you say in your brochures is true is both a selling point and a defence in the event of a misunderstanding.

The following list, and Figure 32, summarise the sort of information parents want. Does the nursery:

- have a formal management structure with clearly defined responsibilities and levels of accountability?
- define its responsibilities with each parent?
- have a system for monitoring progress and adherence to contracts?
- have a procedures manual setting out procedures and standards?
- use standard letters and other documentation?
- have papers that contain evidence of systems and procedures of review?
- have files that contain evidence of management review and approval?
- consult a second senior in areas of difficulty?
- have evidence of such consultations?

If you consider that when a parent is shown around the nursery, answers are given only to the group of questions in Figure 32, it may reassure parents even further about your service if you also offer them answers to the questions in the above list.

Quality assurance and management

Quality assurance is about meeting parents' requirements. It is concerned with management of the service to provide a high probability that the objectives will be achieved. It is not about the

FIRST IMPRESSIONS

- Am I and my child made welcome?
- Are children with special needs made welcome?
- Does it seem that enough warm, individual attention is given to each child?
- Do the children look happy?
- Do they play and talk together?
- Do the children talk with the adults?
- Do the adults listen carefully and give thoughtful replies?
- Do the adults talk to the babies as well as to the older children?
- Are there plenty of toys, books and play equipment, including dressing-up clothes and a home corner, set out for the children to use?
- Are activities such as sand, water, clay and paint also regularly provided?
- Is there enough space for both active and quiet play (a) indoors and (b) outdoors?
- Are there special facilities for babies?

WHAT ABOUT STAFF?

- Are enough adults working with the children?
- Are they trained for the job?
- Do they seem to enjoy being with the children?
- Do they give the children opportunities to make choices and help them to be independent?
- Do they help to build the children's self-confidence with plenty of praise and encouragement?

DAY-TO-DAY

- Do the activities take into account my child's (a) age, (b) cultural background, and (c) special needs?
- Are the activities varied and imaginative – do they stimulate the children to think and talk about them?
- Are both girls and boys encouraged to use all the equipment?
- Is the food good and varied?
- Does the cooking take account of different cultural backgrounds?
- Are mealtimes enjoyed by all the children?

HYGIENE AND SAFETY

- Are the premises kept clean, well maintained and safe?
- Do they have adequate fire appliances?
- Are all heaters and power points protected?
- Are gates and fences secure?
- Is the equipment kept clean, in good repair and safe?
- Are there clear procedures for emergency medical treatment?

Figure 32. Questions that parents focus on when first visiting the nursery.

childcare and philosophy. It entails the establishment of a suitable level of performance and the application of professional skills to the tasks undertaken. Quality management is sound practice.

In 1990, the Department of Health (DoH) undertook research to assess how effective such an approach would be to complement the Children Act in lifting quality. It was generally concluded that it was not the right time for such a formal approach, given that the market was, and still is, largely made up of individual owner-managed nurseries, and the system would be both time-consuming and costly. The government's voucher scheme, however, has brought with it a formal self-appraisal process, required for validation as a voucher-redeeming institution, which is a further push towards quality assurance for parents.

The Department for Education and Employment (DFEE) published its Self-Assessment Schedule in January 1996, which is sent to all provider applicants to the voucher scheme, with the primary purpose of helping them to decide whether they can work towards the education learning outcomes and provide the quality assurance required. It is intended that by working through the schedule a provider will be able to:

- assess whether it can provide nursery education as defined by the DFEE;
- prepare an educational programme and information for parents;
- review its staffing, staff development, management and practice;
- develop its policies for special educational needs (SEN), equal opportunities, children's welfare and relationships with parents;
- meet the requirements of final validation for voucher redemption.

It is not the intention to prescribe a single quality management system for every nursery's practice. That would defeat the objective of motivating nurseries to think about their own activities and objectives. It is for the individual nursery to develop operating methods in which they have confidence and the ability to satisfy parents about their capabilities. Here we address management matters in terms of good business practice. A nursery's ability to provide assurance about the quality of its services can stem only from systematic control over the particular processes in which it is involved. Such a system would recommend that nurseries periodically carry out internal audits of all matters affecting the quality of the service provided. It is not for the audit to question the professional judgement made, but rather to determine that questions were raised and decisions made and communicated at the appropriate time. The key to a successful management system for any nursery lies in the ability to see that the basis of the process is self-evident through audit, review, feedback and continuous improvement.

Quality management does not need complicated procedures, only sufficient documentation to ensure that roles, responsibilities and relationships are clearly identified and any ambiguity in requirements within the nursery are removed.

Preparation of a quality management system is not something to be rushed. Allow a minimum of 18 months in which to define what the nursery's principal preoccupations are, examine how satisfactorily they are carried out and identify where they could be improved to provide greater confidence in achieving objectives. Draft an improved system, review it with all key staff of the nursery, develop the system and allow time for further review before trying it out under controlled conditions. Set realistic objectives and verify whether they are achieved. When the nursery's principals are satisfied, then gradually introduce the quality management system throughout the nursery, keeping it under review. The important outcome of this process is a positive attitude towards continuous self-assessment, but you can seek accreditation for having a quality management system from the British Standards Institution (BSI).

Costs will be incurred by the nursery at two levels:

- firstly in preparing an office quality system manual;
- secondly, if the object is to proceed to independent certification in assessment, certification and subsequent monitoring fees.

The outlay in establishing and maintaining a high-quality management system should be recovered by the nursery through increased efficiency and competitiveness.

A consultancy initiative is available under the auspices of the Department of Trade and Industry (DTI) to provide counselling to small-business owners, if you wish to seek BSI accreditation.

Maintaining the system

The quality management system is a dynamic tool to help your nursery operate with confidence. An essential facet of successful business is to keep the systems used under review and appropriate to the nursery's needs.

In a constantly developing world, opportunities and challenges mean that nurseries must continually review their methods to be sure of maintaining viability and to be ahead in the marketplace. All managers of the nursery should be communicating their views and contributing to its development.

Documenting the process is vital, so that compliance to requirements is apparent. It entails good communication, ability to trace decisions taken, and responsibility identification at all stages from the day a child starts at the nursery.

The nursery, by having well-qualified and committed people who enjoy their work and having its own management routines in place, will in effect have started to develop its quality management system. The next step is to understand its process better, how people are able or not able to carry out their work, and to start to formalise the nursery's 'informal' method of working.

Start to get help in understanding what quality management means for your nursery by listening to those who have studied the subject and its application in practice – in the care sector. This means investing in education and training.

The nursery will then be further helped by selecting a small group of people – or even one person, depending on the size of the nursery – who will be trained in helping to develop the quality management system. This person in your nursery will be a 'missionary' to everyone else – so make sure that a good communicator is chosen.

The nursery's manager must bring every member – from the most senior to the most junior – into the evolving process and not rely on a few to understand and implement the system. Not successfully promoting the system throughout the organisation is the commonest cause of failure.

The nursery will then formalise its process, with the minimum of bureaucracy, and consequently have better control over that process so that it can improve it continuously. Quality management and certification for quality assurance will come naturally as a result.

A nursery needs to decide whether it wishes to obtain a third-party certification for BSI accreditation purposes. Even if a nursery decides against this, I am convinced that travelling the route of quality management – getting to know how effectively the nursery functions – is in itself beneficial and productive.

A certificated nursery is licensed to display the National Certification Mark, incorporating the crown, on its business stationery. This provides a public demonstration that its quality management system has been certified by a competent impartial and accredited body. In time the familiarity of the accreditation system will become a valuable marketing aid and achieve international recognition and respect.

Employing Consultants

Consultants are used by organisations and individuals for several reasons. At first sight it may seem strange for a company to employ an outsider to tackle a task that could be done by internal people, and to pay them well to do it, but consider the following reasons:

- Some organisations may not have the necessary expertise amongst their existing staff to solve a specific problem.
- The expertise may be there but the appropriate people may not be able to fit the assignment into their timetables.
- Even if the right people could take on the task, they themselves might recognise that sometimes an outsider can see problems in a new light and bring a fresh perspective to them.
- Company politics may be such that a disinterested outsider's opinion might more acceptable than that of a staff member.
- A third party, such as an organisation's bank, may insist on an impartial view on a particular issue.
- An outsider can be blamed if things go wrong, and thus keep intact the social bonds existing in the organisation.

Approaches to consulting

In an article 'From expertise to contingency: changes in the nature of consulting', Bob Garratt (1981) identified three styles in consulting practice: expertise consulting, process consulting, and contingency consulting. Each of these is distinct and, if appropriate for the circumstances, equally valid. It is important to know in which area the consultant is operating as the skills needed for each are different.

Expertise consulting

One use of the 'expertise consulting' approach is when an acknowledged expert in a specific area is asked into an organisation to provide a solution to an already identified problem; for example, the need to design and install a wordprocessing system or a new accounting system. In such a case the consultant's main contact is with the person who asked him or her in to look at the problem – you.

This approach may also take the form of a training course where the expert will pass on knowledge or skills to a staff group, either in-house or on a public programme. Once the course is completed, the consultant will not usually have any further contact with the participants. A good trainer can pass on valuable knowledge and skills, but clearly it is what happens afterwards, within the staff team, that matters most.

In his later work, Bob Garratt has likened this approach to surgery; that is, an operation that gives an immediate result, but which cannot always be guaranteed to provide a permanent solution to the problem. It is a drastic, often irreversible, step, because new knowledge is acquired by some individuals, who will undoubtedly want to develop, and others may not be so ready.

Process consulting

Process consulting provides a balance to the logical, rational and often arms-length style of expertise consulting. It involves people much more in their social processes – that is, the feelings and behaviours concerned with a range of managerial problem-solving processes. They often experience a release of energy previously unknown to them.

Working with the emotions in this way may also go beyond the brief envisaged by the manager, and leave the participants fired up with ideas, and with confidence and enthusiasm that the organisation cannot control or accommodate back at the workplace. The relationship between the consultant and the problem-owners becomes quite close during the time they are working together. This can sometimes work against the interests of the organisation as a whole if the participants become alienated from the consultant.

Rather than surgery, this style of consulting may be compared to therapy. As such, it usually needs a complementary approach to enable the participants to develop their newly discovered potential in coping with the 'real' world of their nursery and the problems they face.

Contingency consulting

The aim of the contingency consultant is to become redundant as quickly as possible. This contradicts the conviction held by some that consultants are in business to maximise their fees. The contingency consultant endeavours to make optimal use of the resources already held in an organisation in the form of its staff and their experience. As Bob Garratt writes:

'It attempts to integrate the expertise and process practices when appropriate to the progression of the organisation's problem . . . relying on the asking of high-quality questions and developing an information based approach to problem solving.'

The contingency consultant, whether internal or external, is neither surgeon nor therapist and is used rarely, like small doses of homoeopathic medicine given only when needed.

It may seem strange that, in using a consultant to help solve a problem, the manager is not buying the expert knowledge of the subject to unravel the problem, but rather his or her intelligence and naivety. In many situations, the issues that look like technical puzzles (yet which cannot be solved by staff) are symptoms of a managerial problem. In this case, therefore, finding the solution often depends on the ability to reframe the question in such a way that the nursery's values are made explicit.

Whichever consulting approach is used – expertise, process or contingency – the test of its quality is whether the manager feels at the end of the exercise that the relationship has been one of colleagues acting in a participative way to resolve organisational issues.

Using Advisers

Managing a nursery is a complex and multidisciplinary task. There will be many areas of concern that you can deal with to an extent, and at which you will become accomplished through experience. However, it is critical to be able to identify the point at which specialist help is both prudent and expedient, and to recognise that this will need to be sought externally. This is the start of your business network, your means of maintaining professional contacts and support.

Advisers are so important to the smooth running of a business, however small, that it is vital to employ the right ones. This means not only those who are qualified and experienced enough to do a competent job for you, but also those you like and feel comfortable working with.

The bank manager

'Train your bank manager' was one of the first pieces of advice I was given as an owner of a small business. Even though you may not own the nursery, and accounts may not be your responsibility, you are the public face of the business, and the bank will have greater confidence in the nursery if there are open lines of communication with you.

It certainly is worth making an effort to spend time deciding where to base your account and in getting to know your manager. While the bank nearest to you is the most convenient, it may not be suitable for all your needs. For example, a local branch with little experience of small businesses might not provide all the services you would expect, although a far-sighted manager in such a branch may well be very willing to accommodate you and add a little variety to his or her life. A very large branch in a busy city centre may not be prepared to devote what you consider to be the appropriate attention to your comparatively small interests unless it offers specialist advice and services to small businesses.

Therefore, weigh up the advantages and disadvantages of size, personal attention, specialist services and ease of access when choosing a bank. Talk to the bank manager before you place your business account, even if you have banked there personally for years, and discuss the special needs of a nursery. Find out what sort of information the manager will need from you to keep him or her happy; for example, regular cash-flow forecasts as reassurance that, although there may not be much money in your account at the moment, it will be coming in. If you are going to be away for an unusually long time, or if you are expecting a particularly large bill, let the manager know. Do not let the bank be faced with any unpleasant surprises, because bank managers like to know what is going on, and will probably send you costly letters if they do not.

The role of banks has changed dramatically over the past few years. They now offer a wide range of services, many of which are specifically designed for small businesses. So ask questions, and make sure that you know exactly what the bank can do for you. Handle the bank manager as you would a parent – listen to what he or she needs from you, provide it with alacrity, and the manager in turn should look after you. Bank managers can also be a useful source of new parents – provided, of course, that they have a high regard to you and your nursery.

The accountant

Make sure that you work with a properly qualified accountant who will be able to give you advice on tax-related affairs and on preparing a business plan. The accountant should be consulted about how to prepare and submit profit-and-loss accounts, balance sheets, and cash-flow forecasts. This information may also be available from your bank manager.

Bookkeeping services may be provided by an accountant or you may go to an independent bookkeeper. Some nursery managers keep their own books and submit them to the accountant at the end of the financial year for their professional attention and completion. This takes more self-discipline as you really should do the accounts every day rather than wait to complete the books at the end of the year.

A lawyer

Whoever looks after your legal affairs must be a specialist in small business, who will understand the particular issues affecting nurseries. You will not need to use a lawyer's services in setting up as a sole trader, but it would be wise to employ one if you are entering a partnership agreement. If you take the step of becoming a limited company, your legal adviser will obviously play an important part in helping you avoid all the potential pitfalls of commercial law.

Should you become involved in writing contracts for your parents, or if any parents prepare their own, perhaps on behalf of their employer, you will wish to have them drawn up or checked by someone who specialises in contract law. This may be the same person who looks after your other interests. If not, it may be another lawyer within the same practice, or one who is recommended by your usual adviser. There are now legal practices that specialise in standard contracts for payment of, for example, nursery fees. They will also collect debts and take action on your behalf. It is worth using them.

You may also be involved in drawing up or reviewing terms of employment. This area of law is currently moving very quickly, with new European directives almost daily. It is a specialist area, and legal advice should be chosen accordingly.

Again, establishing a good relationship with your legal adviser is important as, on the few (we hope) occasions when you will work together, speed and cooperation may be of the essence.

An insurance broker

You could draw up your own insurance portfolio by reading all the journals in the local library, but it would take a great deal of time. The safest approach is to go to an adviser, and in the UK there are two types to choose from. There are 'appointed agents' and 'independent financial advisers' (IFAs,) and no one person can have a dual role.

Appointed agents represent one insurance company and they can sell the products only of that company. If the company does not have the full range of products, the agent is not allowed to sell you one that is unsuitable. In the UK these agents must be members of the Life Assurance Unit Trust Regulatory Organisation (LAUTRO).

Independent financial advisers can recommend only the product that is best for you. They must be impartial and must give 'best advice'. IFAs in the UK are usually members of the Financial Intermediaries, Managers and Brokers Regulatory Association (FIMBRA) and the big firms may become registered with the Securities Investment Board direct.

Other sources of insurance advice are the banks and building societies, both of which may be tied to one insurance company. Solicitors and accountants belong to recognised professional bodies and do not have to be governed by FIMBRA or LAUTRO. Some large firms of accountants have set up their own insurance arm and others will be able to introduce you to an IFA.

My experience is that, as with most other purchases, you get what you pay for. The cheapest policy is unlikely to have such broad cover as others. However, you will need advice on calculating the real risks you are facing, and matching a policy to your needs.

There are many 'composite' insurance policies on the market for nurseries and schools, all of which cover the requirements of the Children Act 1989. Optional extras are usually available to cover, for example, non-payment of fees, professional negligence, and staff sickness.

Bibliography

Constable, J. and McCormick, R. (1987) *The Making of British Managers*. London: BIM/CBI.

Handy, C. (1987) *The Making of Managers*. London: HMSO.

Leach, P. (1994) *Children First*. London: Penguin.

Moss, P. and Melhuish, E. (eds) (1991) *Current Issues in Day Care for Young Children*. London: HMSO.

National Children's Bureau (1991) *Young Children in Group Day Care: Guidelines for Good Practice*. London: NCB.

Penn, H. and Riley, K. (1992) *Managing Services for the Under Fives*. Harlow: Longman.

Pugh, G., De'Att, E. and Smith, C. (1994) *Confident Parents, Confident Children*. London: National Children's Bureau.

Rodd, G. (1994) *Leadership in Early Childhood*. Buckingham: Open University Press.

Rumbold, A. (1990) *Starting with Quality: Report of the Committee of Inquiry into the Educational Experiences Offered to Three- and Four-Year-Olds*. London: HMSO for the Department of Education and Science.

Social Services Inspectorate (1995) *Inspection of Private and Voluntary Day Nurseries for Children Under Eight: Overview Report*. London: Department of Health.

Sylva, K. (1994) The impact of early learning on children's later development. Ball, C. (ed.) In: *The Importance of Early Learning*. London: Royal Society for the Encouragement of the Arts, Manufacturing and Commerce.

Vernon, J. and Smith, C. (1994) *Day Nurseries at a Crossroads*. London: National Children's Bureau.

References

Ashridge Strategic Management Centre, London.

Bettleheim, B. (1987) *A Good Enough Parent*. Thames and Hudson.

Carlisle, H. M. (1979) *Management Essentials: Concepts and Applications*. Chicago: Science Research Associates Inc.

Childcare Association (1991) *Code of Practice*. London: Childcare Association.

Cohen, B. (1990) *Caring for Children*. London: Family Policy Studies Centre.

Department for Education and Employment (1996) *Nursery Education Scheme*. London: HMSO.

Department of Health (1991) *The Children Act 1989: Guidance and Regulations,* volume 2. London: HMSO.

Early Childhood Education Forum (1996) *Quality in Diversity*. London: ECEF.

Garratt, R. (1981) *From expertise to contingency: changes in the nature of consulting*. In: Management, Education and Development (workshop), volume 12, part II.

Garratt, R. (1990) *Creating a Learning Organisation*. Cambridge: Fitzwilliam Publishing.

Goldschmied, E. and Jackson, S. (1994) *People Under Three*. London: Routledge.

Handy, C. (1987) *The Making of Managers*. London: HMSO.

Hodgkinson, C. (1991) *Education leadership*. In: The Moral Art. Albany: State University of New York Press.

Hogg, C. and Harker, L. (1992) *The Family Friendly Employer*. London: Daycare Trust.

Inner London Education Authority (1980) *Junior School Project*. London: ILEA.

Katz, A. (1994) *The family is fine . . . but under pressure*. In: Sainsburys Magazine. London: New Crane Publishing Ltd.

Leach, P. (1994) *Children First*. London: Penguin.

Moss, P. and Pence, A. (1994) *Valuing Quality in Early Childhood Services*. London: Paul Chapman.

National Children's Bureau (1991) *Young Children in Group Day Care: Guidelines for Good Practice*. London: NCB.

National Commission on Education (1993) *Learning to Succeed.* London: NCE.

Pascal, C. (1990) *Under Fives in Infant Classrooms.* Stoke-on-Trent, Trentham Press.

Peat Marwick (1990), London.

Pedler, M., Boydell, T., Burgoyne, J. (1989) *Towards the Learning Company.* In: Management, Education and Development, volume 20, part I.

Penn, H. and Riley, K. (1992) *Managing Services for the Under Fives.* Harlow: Longman.

Pre-School Playgroups (1994) *Accreditation Scheme* (Now called Pre-School Learning Alliance). London: PSP.

Rodd, G. (1994) *Leadership in Early Childhood.* Buckingham: Open University Press.

Rumbold, A. (1990) *Starting with Quality: Report of the Committee of Inquiry into the Educational Experiences Offered to Three- and Four-Year-Olds.* London: HMSO for the Department of Education and Science.

Schools Curriculum Assessment Authority (1996) *Desirable Learning Outcomes for Children.* London: SCAA.

Sylva, K. (1994) The impact of early learning on children's later development. In: Ball, C. (ed.), *The Importance of Early Learning.* London: Royal Society for the Encouragement of the Arts, Manufacturing and Commerce.

Thomas Coram Research Unit (1996) *Group Day Care.* London: TCRU.

Vernon, J. and Smith, C. (1994) *Day Nurseries at a Crossroads.* London: National Children's Bureau.

Whitebook, M., Howes, C. and Phillips, D. (1989) *The National Childcare Staffing Study.* Oakland, USA.

Whittaker, P. (1995) Nursery World Conference; Olympia, London.

Worcester College of Higher Education (1994) *Effective Early Learning Project.* Worcester: WC.

Useful Addresses

Childcare and Education Association,
407 Coppergate House,
16 Brune Street,
London E1 7NJ

National Children's Bureau,
8 Wakley Street,
London EC1V 7QE

British Institute of Management,
The Institute of Management,
Management House,
Cottingham Road,
Corby

Women in Management,
64 Marryat Road,
London SW19

Index

Note: page references in *italics* refer to figures and tables.